Too Tired To Cook

The Shift Worker's Guide To Working
(and Surviving) In A 24/7 World

Audra Starkey

BALBOA.
PRESS

A DIVISION OF HAY HOUSE

Balboa Press books may be ordered through booksellers or by contacting:

Balboa Press
A Division of Hay House
1663 Liberty Drive
Bloomington, IN 47403
www.balboapress.com.au
1 (877) 407-4847

Print information available on the last page.

ISBN: 978-1-5043-1875-4 (sc)
ISBN: 978-1-5043-1876-1 (e)

Balboa Press rev. date: 08/01/2019

"Shift Work:
Unless you've worked it yourself,
you can never gain a
true appreciation
of just how hard it is."

–Audra Starkey

Dedication

This book is dedicated to you, my fellow shift worker, who gets up tirelessly and goes into work every day while others are still sound asleep in bed. And no matter where you are in the world or what line of work you're in, you are most likely plagued with overwhelming feelings of exhaustion, disillusionment, and poor health due to the irregular hours you work.

Quite simply, you are doing what most people would not, or could not do, often at the expense of your own health.

If the quote on the previous page resonated, rest assured, you are not alone. After sharing it on my Healthy Shift Worker Facebook page a few years ago, it generated over 4 million organic views, 42,000 shares, 19,000 likes, and over 1,000 comments.

It quite literally took on a life of its own, to a point where forty thousand people from around the world decided to share it too. To put this into context, that's the capacity of the entire Gabba (a cricket and football stadium in my hometown of Brisbane, Australia).

So despite what others may tell you, shift work is not easy. It's hard. Really hard.

Incredibly, according to the Australian Bureau of Statistics (2015), almost two million Australians work shift work, along with 20 percent of the world's workforce. This equates to nearly 0.7 billion workers worldwide, which represents an enormous part of the global economy [1] [2].

Quite simply, we need shift workers, but more importantly, we need you to be healthy.

It's why I wrote this book: to provide you with some help and guidance when others may put you in the too-hard basket and tell you to just quit your job.

Instead, I've got a better idea. Why don't we focus on educating ourselves around shift work health? Focusing on solutions; tips and strategies to support you, which is exactly what this book does.

So from one shift worker to another, I want to help you to tackle this shift-working role the best way you can because most people don't want to quit; they just want to learn how to become the healthiest versions of themselves, despite working 24/7.

Audra

Contents

Foreword xi
Cyndi O'Meara xi
Tracey Rohweder...xv

Part 1. Introduction

A Date with Destiny..2
How This Book Came About..6

Part 2. Welcome!

Why Reading This Book Could Save Your Life (and
Relationships) 14
Why Too Tired to Cook? 23

Part 3. The Struggles Are Real, and How to Manage Them

Struggle 1: Ongoing and Relentless Sleep Deprivation and
Disruption 28
Struggle 2: My Uniform Must Be Shrinking - Weight
Fluctuations and an Expanding Waistline...................................... 51
Struggle 3: Feelings of Stress, Anxiety, and Depression 69
Struggle 4: A Depleted and Burnt-Out Immune System..............90

Struggle 5: A Disrupted Family and Social Life, Strained
Relationships, and Tension in the Workplace 102

Part 4. Conclusion

Where to from Here? The Choice Is Up to You 114
Healthy Shift Worker Checklist 117

Part 5. Healthy Shift Worker Recipes

Energising Early Shift Recipes 120
Nourishing Night Shift Recipes 125
Curb Sugar-Cravings 135

Special Thanks 143
References 147
About Audra Starkey 161

Foreword
Cyndi O'Meara

I studied anthropology at the University of Colorado where I learnt how the foods we ate over the thousands of generations of culture and tradition enabled survival of the human race. Our adaptation to climate and food were all about ancient wisdom passed down through the generations.

My focus has always been food, but over the decades I've learnt that food was not the only ingredient that helped in the survival of the human race. Sunlight, sleep, water, connection and magnetism to name a few, were all important for existence and perpetuation of the human species.

Life was simpler then. You went to bed when the sun went down and got up when it rose; There was no scheduled work day - you weren't isolated at a desk staring at a screen all hours of the day and night. The TV didn't exist so time was spent with loved ones communicating and telling stories. Cars were not a thing so walking was the only mode of transport. The only stress was if there was a predator nearby where you had to make a decision to flee or fight – the stress was but an instant in time, not a whole year of pressure. All the things that were needed for human health mentally and physically were at our finger tips; we naturally lived in a rhythm of life.

Enter 2019.

Wifi, EMFs, smart phones, social media, poor diet, chemical

agriculture, overburden of chemicals, continuous stress, sleepless nights, climate change, all-nighters, lighting to keep you awake, stimulants, medications, no sun, no exercise and basically all the things that our evolutionary body has never had to handle. Throw in shift work and all that comes with it and our evolutionary bodies fail to thrive, unless we become aware and make changes to rectify the situation.

We don't have modern bodies that can deal with these enormous modern day changes, but rather we have evolutionary bodies that need the right ingredients in order to be well, energetic and vibrant.

Think of it this way. A plant needs sunlight, water, soil and nutrients in order to grow and thrive and if it is a food-bearing tree, it needs these ingredients to produce its produce. Take these elements away and it will wilt and die. We also need ingredients that will help our evolutionary body thrive - sunlight, sleep, food, water and connection are the fundamentals. If we are not thinking about these important elements, we fail to recognise all the aspects that may be causing physical and mental illness.

Our evolutionary body has adapted to night and day, sunlight and darkness, real foods and movement. Our circadian rhythms are not just about sleep and waking but they also dictate many systems in our body including the endocrine system, blood system (including the heart), brain and nervous system, digestive system, musculoskeletal system and the immune system. In other words, our circadian rhythms are the body's master clock that is set by the rising and setting sun.

Thank goodness our bodies are forgiving and resilient! Do the wrong thing by it by eating junk, having a screen in front of your eyes at night, a lack of sleep, not drinking water and not exercising and you will probably get sick. Change those parameters and the body will, in most cases, bounce back.

Audra Starkey in this wonderful book Too Tired to Cook addresses action steps for the shift worker to take, but these are not only for shift workers. We all need to hear these messages; they are simple strategies that support the evolutionary body.

Audra's book is concise, impactful, filled with referenced facts and quick, easy recipes – it has all the ingredients you need in order to support your evolutionary body to health and vitality. This book could turn the tide of research that shows the negative health impact of shift work.

Awareness is the first part of this education. Once you know the issues and problems then the solutions are in action steps in this book. Following this book step by step, action by action, will help you survive your shift working days.

Happy changing shift working habits.

Cyndi O'Meara
Nutritionist, Speaker, Author of Changing Habits Changing Lives
Founder of Changing Habits
Founder of The Nutrition Academy
Producer of the Documentary *What's with Wheat?*

Foreword

Tracey Rohweder

I stumbled across Audra, aka The Healthy Shift Worker, on Facebook about five years ago. Since then, the HSW movement has gone from strength to strength.

Having been a shift worker for more than twelve years, I couldn't believe my luck when I found someone out there who seemed to understand what I was going through and how tough this gig can be. But more importantly, someone who really cares about what she does. It's why I jumped at the chance to come in and see her in the student client when the opportunity arose.

Of course, I knew Audra had an interest in shift work, but what I didn't expect was to meet a lady SO passionate, dedicated and enthusiastic about this non-traditional work life. We clicked straight away. We were on the same page. And I am beyond proud this amazing person has become a dear friend.

It was like she was inside my head (probably a scary place Audra!) and 100% knew the struggles that come with working a 24/7 roster. She is supportive, empathetic and dedicated to helping shift workers live a better life. Her passion is unwavering. Her message is consistent. She genuinely wants to help people improve their quality of life. And in the pages that follow, she gives real-life, easy-to-achieve tips for the time-poor and sleep-deprived.

And if you are a shift worker – that's you!

While reading the book, I laughed more times than I can remember. There were lots of virtual high fives and calling out "Yes!", "Wow," and "That's me!!", much to the amusement of my cats. Audra's humorous anecdotes, her experiences, and her ability to keep it real are the keys to her success in translating her face-to-face presentations to the page.

To anyone who is working shift work – you NEED this book (#gamechanger). The contents of these pages could change your life. Without a doubt, they have changed mine for the better.

If you have an equally challenging job of supporting a shift worker (we couldn't do it without you!) then PLEASE read this book. It's going to open your eyes to our world and give you some insights as to why we are like we are. And then, share with your shift worker and those around you.

Audra, I am incredibly proud of you and the heartfelt words in this book. I can't wait to see HSW take on the world and be a voice for the shift workers globally!

Tracey Rohweder
Shift Worker seventeen years; wife of a Shift Worker; Mum to two teens, two cats and a dog; – and a Healthy Shift Worker Fan Girl.

Part 1.
Introduction

A Date with Destiny

"Family is not just those who share your blood;
it's those who you share your life with."
— Unknown

SEPTEMBER 17, 2014, is a day I will never forget. It was an unusually quiet morning at the airport, a workplace which had become my home away from home for over half my life since commencing my career in aviation way back in 1993, at the tender age of twenty-two. The usual buzz and frenzy of a busy airport environment suddenly became still and motionless, as I was ushered into the airport duty manager's office and politely asked to take a seat.

While I had a bit of an idea of what was about to happen, I had a feeling that whatever was about to unfold between these four walls in the next few minutes had the potential to change the direction of my life forever.

And it did.

As I sat nervously across the desk looking directly into the eyes of the manager who was on shift at the time, he began with the words, "Audra, I've got some good news for you."

I smiled back at him across the table.

"I'm happy to advise you've been successful in your application for voluntary redundancy. Your last date with Qantas will be on October 28, 2014."

What did he say? Did I hear correctly? "My last day with Qantas will be when?"

My head began to spin as the words echoed through my head, and I tried to absorb what had just happened.

To my surprise, the first words which came out of my mouth were "Can I give you a hug?"

He looked back across the table at me, somewhat puzzled, stirred in his seat, and politely replied, "Um, well, I don't know you that well."

He was right. He didn't know me that well, as he'd only been appointed the position just a few months earlier.

But right at that very moment, I just really needed a hug.

You see, little did this guy know, I was about to take a huge leap of faith and walk away from the only career that I'd ever really known, to embark on an entirely different profession that I hoped one day would change the lives of millions of people around the world, that being shift workers.

In order to make this happen, it meant that I was about to close the door on nearly two decades of working 24/7, which I have to say has been one hell of a crazy rollercoaster ride filled with fun and euphoric moments, mixed together with mentally, emotionally, and physically exhausting ones.

That's because throughout my career, I'd worked shifts that started at 3 a.m. to the opposite end of the spectrum, where I would start at 8:30 p.m. and finish at the ungodly hour of 4:30 a.m.

You name it, and I've worked it.

And to anyone who's ever worked shift work before, you will know how incredibly tough and, at times, downright exhausting this can be.

Not only are these feelings of constant fatigue and tiredness an incredibly hard and unforgiving way to live, but it can also be a lonely ride, as we often feel as though we're some weird nocturnal animal working through the night and into the early hours of the morning.

So September 17 is a date that will be forever etched into my memory, as will October 28, 2014, the very last day of my shift-working career in an industry that I loved. It was a day which was filled with mixed emotions, as I voluntarily closed the door on my shift-working career and said goodbye to my shift-working family, which was probably the most heart-wrenching decision of all.

> *Saying goodbye to my shift working family was the most heart-wrenching decision of all.*

One of the biggest things I've learned over the years from working in a shift-working environment is that family is not only those who we are related to by blood; it's those we share our life with, which of course includes our workmates too.

Ironically, this is what makes working shift work so unique. It allows us to develop a much deeper connection with our colleagues as a result of spending so much family time together, including weekends and holidays, like Easter and Christmas, to name just two.

So considering shift work can often be an incredibly lonely and thankless occupation, our shift-working family can often be the glue that holds us together.

And that, of course, includes you: the reason I've written this book and the driving force behind going back to university at the tender age of thirty-nine to learn all I could about nutrition and shift work health.

But I'll share more about that shortly.

Right now, I want you to know that you're not alone in your struggles with working these crazy and irregular hours, and I'm here to help.

In the following pages, I'm going to share some of my shift-working insights and wisdom, and let you know that despite the craziness of your sleep-deprived world, there is light at the end of the tunnel. All I ask is that you be prepared to shift your mindset a little and be open to what you're about to read.

As a fellow shift worker, I want to reach out to you and say, "I know it's hard, but you're going to be okay," just as I would say to any member of my family because in my eyes, we are the same.

To your good health,

Audra x

How This Book Came About

NOW I'M GOING to assume if you've gone to the trouble of purchasing this book (thank you for doing that, by the way), then you've had times when you've asked yourself, "Can I keep doing this? Can I keep working these crazy and irregular hours?"

I know I did, many times.

That niggling question pretty much led me down a very long and winding path, trying to make sense of what is, hands down, one of the most challenging occupations on the planet.

Ironically, this continual quest for answers turned me into a bit of an accidental expert on shift work health, not only because I spent years working shift work myself, but as a result of working exclusively with shift working clients one-on-one while studying to become a nutritionist.

My passion and dedication to shift work health even led one of my lecturers at university say to me, during the final semester of my nutritional medicine degree, "Audra, I think you care too much for shift workers."

"Audra, I think you care too much for shift workers."

As a former shift worker and soon-to-be health care practitioner, I found this comment quite perplexing and to a degree, quite hurtful. Thankfully, it gave me even more drive and motivation to write and publish the book you're now holding.

So let me share with you exactly how this book came to fruition.

I began shift work when I was twenty-two years old and walked away from it when I was forty-three. Apart from a couple of years of working "normal person hours," for eighteen years, I lived and breathed shift work. I also spent many of those years trying to navigate my way through what felt like a thick, murky shift-work fog. Metaphorically speaking, it was like walking in a tunnel, holding a dimly lit torch and not being able to see the hurdles and hazards ahead. I'm sure you can relate.

The real catalyst, however, came about eight months after my workplace, in their very wisdom, decided to undergo some massive changes (without consulting the staff). Think procedural changes, restructuring, policy revisions, and roster changes which included split days off. You name it, it was all happening, and with very little consideration to the fatigue-inducing effects that it was having on every member of staff.

I came home from a particularly crazy and hectic shift one day, removed my shoes, and proceeded to curl up into a ball on the floor of our bedroom.

I told Dale, my husband, "I can't do this anymore. I just can't."

I'd reached a point of burn out.

I was physically, mentally, and emotionally exhausted.

Every muscle in my body ached from top to toe, I could hardly string two words together because my sleep-deprived brain was in a complete fog, and I became overwhelmed with emotion when Dale wrapped his supportive arms around me, triggering an outpouring of tears down my face.

I felt so lost, so overwhelmed, and I had no idea what to do.

> I felt so lost, so overwhelmed, and had no idea what to do.

While my beautiful husband told me to "just quit," I wasn't ready to walk away from a job that I had enjoyed for so many years, just like that.

I'd also already gone through an incredibly stressful time a few years earlier, when I lost my job with Ansett Australia, the country's second major domestic airline carrier at the time when it went into voluntary receivership, leaving over sixteen thousand people unemployed, including myself.

Realistically, throwing in the towel and quitting my job was not an option, anyway. Like most young couples, we had a mortgage and bills to pay, and I also didn't feel right about placing this entire financial burden on my husband.

While I would often come home feeling utterly exhausted, thanks to the sleep-deprived lifestyle, I still genuinely loved my job and wasn't ready to hang up my alarm clock for good … just yet.

What I needed was some help, someone to tell me, "I know it's hard, Audra, but you're going to be okay."

But there was no one.

No one to put my mind at rest and tell me that I was going to be okay or to help me navigate some of the hurdles we face while working 24/7, all whilst keeping my sanity too.

So I went looking for answers. I went searching for that one book that was going to provide me with practical and straightforward solutions which addressed the many struggles we face when working 24/7, things like sleep deprivation, weight fluctuations, having no energy to exercise, stress, a disrupted family and social life, and more.

In essence, I wanted to hear from someone who understood me, someone who got me, had walked in my shoes, and was therefore suitably qualified to give me the advice I was desperately searching for.

But this book did not exist.

Despite scrolling through countless books on weight loss, nutrition, and exercise (let's face it: there are millions of these), I was totally amazed (and somewhat disheartened) to discover nothing had been written specifically to help shift workers.

Now and then, I would get a little excited when I found something close, but my excitement would soon wane after realising the author had never actually worked shift work, so didn't really get me at all.

I also became increasingly frustrated whenever I'd pick up a book on sleep. Why? Because almost every book written on the subject recommended two things:

1. Go to bed when you feel sleepy.
2. Get out of bed at the same time every day.

Pfft! Really?

I couldn't help but laugh out loud when I read a book which suggested not using an alarm clock. I'm not quite sure how we would get to work on time without these trusty little gadgets, especially for those rather hideous 3 a.m. starts!

I even remember a time early into my career, when I slept through *two* alarm clocks because I was so tired and exhausted. It made me ponder the idea of inventing an alarm clock which had an extendable hand that reaches out and shakes you to wake you up. A bestseller, I'm sure.

All in all, few of the books I've read on sleep have been helpful, given we have to get up at an ungodly hour.

"Not sleeping is bad for us," they say. "We should stick to a regular sleep routine," they say; blah, blah, blah. Some books even recommended that we quit shift work altogether. Hmmm. Although this would undeniably improve our health and well-being, realistically, the world would come to a complete standstill if we didn't have shift workers.

Think air travel, emergency services, hospitality, manufacturing. I could go on and on. So even though quitting may be a great way to improve our health, it's probably not a viable option for the majority of people who are reading this book right now.

> *The world would come to a standstill if we didn't have shift workers.*

I also know plenty of shift workers who love their jobs but just need a little guidance to manage their health. Unfortunately, more often than not, we get put into the "too-hard" basket by many well-intentioned health care practitioners because they quite literally don't know what to do with us.

The majority of companies who employ shift workers, also, quite incredibly, fail to offer their staff any type of induction or ongoing training around the topic of shift work health. It's what ultimately led to the development of my signature Healthy Shift Worker Workplace Wellness Seminars that I now deliver for organisations all over Australia.

But I digress.

So after my relentless search for that one book, all those years ago, I soon realised that it was going to be up to me. I was going to have to start educating myself and find a way to stay healthy so that I could then share all I learned with others.

From the words of Toni Morrison: "If there's a book that you want to read, but it hasn't been written yet: then you MUST write it."

So I did.

After years of research, combined with a whole lot of personal experience, along with going back to school at the age of thirty-nine, *Too Tired to Cook* is the book that many shift workers have been searching for but have been unable to find.

I'm most proud of this book because it's written by a shift worker, for a shift worker. After spending two decades working 24/7, I do get it, and I want you to know that I really do care.

So for me, this is personal. I went through many of the struggles I talk about in this book but was unable to find anyone who could give me practical (and sustainable) advice to help me to get the results I was looking for.

> *This book has been written by a shift worker, for a shift worker.*

It's why I've dedicated the last ten years of my life to learn all I can to help all those who work 24/7.

While leaving my aviation career, the only profession I ever really knew, was an incredibly tough and at times frightening decision, I knew I had to take a leap of faith because there was no one out there helping shift workers. So after many hours, days, weeks, months, and years, that leap of faith has finally materialised in the form of this book. I sincerely hope you gain lots of valuable information to help you to become the best version of yourself whilst working 24/7.

Who This Book Is For

This book was written specifically for those who work (or plan to work) shift work, along with those whose partner works shift work. In other words, if you (or someone you love) have never worked shift work before, or have no plans on working it, then this book won't really make much sense to you.

That being said, if you have friends and family members who are shift workers and you want to gain a better understanding of why they may act or behave the way they do, then I definitely recommend you read it from cover to cover.

If you are a health care practitioner that has shift working clients, then I urge you to read this book too, or at the very least, recommend it to your clients. As I highlighted at the beginning, unless you've worked shift work yourself, you can never truly understand just how hard it is. But it doesn't necessarily mean we want to quit our jobs altogether. So sharing this book with your clients may be a valuable addition to the treatment plan that you prescribe for them.

Lastly, I'd like to dedicate this book to those individuals who head up shift-working organisations or have some influence on the health and well-being of their shift-working staff, because they're struggling, and this book will help to explain why.

So it's time to push aside all those half-read books that may be gathering dust on your bedside table and replace them with *Too Tired to Cook*. I promise it's going to be one of those books you want to read in its entirety, from start to finish.

Part 2.
Welcome!

Why Reading This Book Could Save Your Life (and Relationships)

---

*"It's much harder to turn a condition around,
than preventing it in the first place."*
-Dr Tom O'Bryan

ONE OF THE most enjoyable parts of my career in aviation was when I worked as a trainer; because deep down, I've always had a yearning to help people. In fact, many members of my family are teachers, including aunts, uncles, and grandparents, so I guess in some way, education has been, and always will be, in my blood. Even my workmates would often say to me that I had the patience of a saint, so I guess that helped too.

However, it wasn't until I had a staff member arrive into my classroom late one day, holding a hamburger, doughnut, and soft drink in hand (and it was only 9 a.m.), that my interest in aviation

14

suddenly switched towards nutrition, or more specifically, shift work health.

This lady was one of those work colleagues that we all love to work with. Always happy, always smiling and often making light-heartedness of a stressful situation, which is why I turned to her with a cheeky smile and said to her, "That's an interesting choice for breakfast!"

Her response to me was, "I've been up since 4 a.m. and in need of some sustenance."

What did she just say? In need of some what?

It was in that moment that I had an epiphany.

It was as if time stood still for a few minutes, as I pondered her reply and reference to a hamburger, doughnut and soft drink as sustenance.

Because something didn't sound quite right with that sentence.

While I'm happy to admit my diet was far from perfect, I always assumed that a hamburger, doughnut, and soft drink was probably not the best choice to nourish my tired and weary body, especially when working 24/7. And especially not at 9am, regardless of our shift.

So when I left work that day, my mind was buzzing and thinking to myself *Why on earth have we never had any training on this? Why have we never been provided with any tips or guidance on how to take care of our health while working irregular hours, given it forms the foundation of our role as a shift worker?*

Fast forward a few years later, and as I approached the ripe old age of forty, I decided to make the courageous (some would say crazy!) decision, to go back to university to obtain a better understanding of how what we eat when working irregular hours, can influence our health for the better, or to its detriment.

It was time to immerse myself and learn all that I could about shift work health, with a special focus around nutrition.

My Journey to Learn About Shift Work Health Begins

When I began studying a Bachelor of Science Degree majoring in Nutritional Medicine back in 2010, my sole reason was to gain a better appreciation of how nutrition can enhance the well-being of shift workers, so that I could then give back to my profession and share all that I had learned.

Now I must admit, I thought all I had to do was learn about the different macro- and micro-nutrients, get my head around some of the biochemical pathways that make us tick, and then put together some healthy recipes and meal plans for shift workers that I could distribute, and voila, I'd be done.

Except that my nutritional medicine journey (or, more specifically, the health science portion of that degree) taught me more than I ever imagined, and I mean way more.

This is because I took every opportunity I could to undertake research and work on assignments that had to do with shift work health. Upon reflection, I'm sure many of my lecturers rolled their eyes each time another assignment came through from me. Whether it had to do with sleep deprivation, stress, a depleted immune system, or hormonal dysregulation (which can occur as a consequence of sleep deprivation), I was on a mission to know and learn more.

> I took every opportunity to undertake research and work on assignments that had to do with shift work health.

However, as I sat glued to my computer, reading research article after research article on various studies and clinical trials undertaken on shift workers, my heart would begin to sink.

Time and time again, the evidence kept showing that shift workers were prone to various chronic health conditions, including gastrointestinal complaints, obesity, insulin resistance, cardiovascular disease, hormonal cancers, and mental health disorders, to name a few.

At first, I found this information incredibly unsettling. Tears would well up in my eyes as I read journal article after journal article, many of which said the same thing. However, those feelings of sadness quickly moved to frustration and then, dare I say, anger. (For those of you who don't know me, it takes a fair bit to ruffle my feathers, but my feathers were starting to become quite ruffled!)

Why? Well, because even though this research is published for anyone to read, who knows about it, or reads it, other than academics or university students like myself?

Who knows about this research or reads it, other than academics or university students like myself?

Prior to 2010, I was a shift worker who had never read a journal article in her life. Why would I? My background wasn't in science; it was in aviation, so I had no need (or desire) to read through a scientific journal article, which often feels like you need to learn another language to understand and decipher it, anyway. Not to mention (no offence to the researchers), they're not exactly the most exciting things to read and can quickly put you to sleep, which is pretty easy to do when you're already running on limited amounts of it.

It was in that moment my journey to improve the health of shift workers took a completely different turn.

It was no longer going to be all about recipes, nutrients, and meal plans.

The more I read and learned, the more I realised the biochemical consequences, on a cellular level, of having to endure disruptive sleep patterns which was having catastrophic effects on our health.

It's the sleep deprivation that is the real driver behind our ill health when we work 24/7.

Because it's the sleep disruption that is the real driver behind our ill health when we work 24/7; the poor diet, lack of exercise, and strained relationships come second. They're a by-product of lack of sleep.

So I made the decision, right there and then, that I needed to refocus a lot of my attention towards sleep, and then share this information with those who needed to know it the most – and that, of course, is you.

As I immersed myself in these journal articles, trying to make sense of what I was reading, I began to take notes on the important bits, the urgent, life-saving bits which I felt were vital for every shift worker to know and understand, so I could one day put it all together in a book, the book you're reading right now.

One thing I want to re-iterate is that, while the research indicates shift workers are prone to developing certain conditions, it's a risk factor not a cause.

If it was a cause, then every single shift worker would be overweight or have insulin resistance, which we know is not the case.

We also have to take into consideration the chicken and the egg. In other words, which one happened first?

Was it the poor diet which led to the type 2 diabetes, or was it the sleep disruption? We all know when we're incredibly tired; our food is often one of the first things to be neglected. However, if we're going to sit down to highly refined and processed meals day after day, month after month, year after year, then poor health is going to be inevitable. That's regardless of whether you work 24/7 or 9–5.

Fortunately, our bodies are very forgiving. They can put up with a lot, but there will come a time when it tells you, "I've had enough." It may be through various physical signs and symptoms, some big and some small, which should not be ignored.

I don't share this information to scare you; it's just about creating awareness, an awareness that, given what you do, you have to endure sleep disruption and work against your natural circadian rhythms. Therefore, you can be prone to specific health conditions.

If anything, just knowing how vulnerable you are to developing ill health and chronic disease as a result of a sleep-disruptive lifestyle should be enough to stir you into action to take better care of your health.

> *Just knowing how vulnerable you are to developing ill health should be enough to stir you into action to take better care of your health.*

It did for me. The more I read, the more conscious I became of my health.

As shift workers, we are subjected to disrupted sleeping patterns, ongoing artificial light exposure, and various other forms of stress the human body is not designed to tolerate, week after week, year after year (if ever).

The harsh reality is that human beings have not adapted to working 24/7 and probably never will. Certainly not in my lifetime, that's for sure.

So this book is designed to provide you with lots of valuable information to reduce your risk factors so you don't become one of the statistics I read about in my six years of university study.

How This Book Was Written

I've tried hard to write this book in a way that is easy to read because I know you're tired. Actually, let's not sugar-coat it. You're exhausted! I think we can all relate to lying on the sofa with a good book, and falling asleep soon after, thanks to a few too many early or night shifts.

That being said, I do delve into the scientific research and jargon now and then because, as a clinically trained nutritionist, evidence-based medicine is an integral part of what I do. I also think it's vital for you to understand the reasons behind my recommendations; when we know why things are the way they are, we're more likely to make better decisions.

So my job is to bring some of this research to you, but in a simple way that anyone can understand.

I'm also an advocate of anecdotal evidence, particularly when it comes to clinical trials and being able to replicate these studies in the real world; this is not always possible, whether due to logistical or financial reasons. We also can't afford to stand around and wait until all the research comes out before we begin to change our behaviour. Your health is important. We need to start doing things differently before we run out of time and miss our opportunity to do so.

> *We can't afford to stand around and wait until all the research comes out before we change our behaviour.*

But Why Haven't You Included XYZ?

There is so much that I could have included in this book, but because reading a book can sometimes make us feel even more tired, I want to ensure I keep your attention from beginning to end. Quite simply, this is one of those books that you do not want to skip chapters. Every single section in this book contains valuable information that is going to help you to improve your health (and relationships), but in a holistic way.

It's about taking a step back and looking at your shift work life in its entirety, the big picture. Because let's face it, it's often the simplest of lifestyle adjustments that can have the most profound impact on our health.

In a nutshell, this book is written in a way to help you to help yourself, because how you take care of your

> *It's often the simplest of lifestyle adjustments that can have the most profound impact on our health.*

health right now, and into the future, can either increase that risk or reduce it substantially.

Will It Save Your Life and Your Relationships?

To be perfectly honest, I have absolutely no idea, but what I do know is that we all have 100 percent control in how we take care of ourselves, from the food we put into our mouth to whether we choose to get off the couch and move our bodies more.

100 percent.

I've also learned over the years from working with clients that common sense is not common practice. We're often searching for some external, complicated reason as to why we may not be the healthiest we can be right now, which in some cases may ring true, but for the majority of us, better health comes from implementing common-sense practices.

For example, taking all the supplements in the world will not improve your sleep, if you continue to be on your mobile devices when you should be sleeping. You're also throwing your hard-earned cash down the drain because constant mobile phone exposure leads to an overstimulation of the nervous system, which interferes with the production of sleep-promoting hormones necessary for rest to occur.

So never underestimate the power of common-sense practices; the simple act of turning your mobile phone off one hour before bedtime can dramatically improve your sleep and, ultimately, your health.

A Final Note

Now before we embark on this journey together, I want you to know that I don't have all of the answers, nor do I pretend to. However, I do have a strong desire to learn, analyse, and educate others, because as the saying goes, we can give people a fish, and they eat for a day, but if you teach them to fish, they eat for a lifetime.

And I don't want you to be healthy, just for a day.

Many people who work shift work often do so for decades at a time, so we need to set you up for long-term success. It means sharing tips and strategies that are both practical and sustainable, that you're going to be able to weave into your shift-working lifestyle, whatever that is for you.

> It's incredibly easy not to look after yourself when working 24/7, but this makes it even more critical that you do.

It's also crucial to acknowledge that it's incredibly easy *not* to take care of yourself when working 24/7, but this makes it even more critical that you do.

My biggest wish is that you don't wait until you're battling a health crisis before you begin to take care of yourself. Let's start to work on ways to improve your health starting from today, because we've only got one body and one chance to take care of it.

"Take care of your body. It's the only place you have to live."
– Jim Rohn.

Why Too Tired to Cook?

I decided to call this book *Too Tired to Cook* because when we work early shifts, night shifts, evening shifts, rotating shifts, and any type of irregular shifts, this is how we feel: too tired to cook.

Not many shift workers feel like whipping up some kind of culinary delight after being up at "stupid o'clock" (a phrase lovingly coined by one of my shift-working clients).

Not me, that's for sure.

Which is why, if you've got your hands on this book right now, I'm pretty confident that you can relate when I say this too-tired-to-cook existence leads to us reaching for quick and easy options, which are not always the healthiest (think two-minute noodles, frozen ready-made meals, and takeaway pizza).

Sounding familiar?

However, I'm going to put my nutritionist hat on now because relying on not-cooked-from-scratch meals can be the beginning of our downfall, as these highly refined and processed foods are not real food.

Sure, they may contain food-like ingredients, but are they real food?

Not even close.

For the most part, our grandparents and great-grandparents wouldn't be able to recognise a lot of the foods we often have to hoover down at an accelerated pace, thanks to our time-allocated meal breaks.

That is, of course, if we even get a designated meal break.

Coupled with eating at all the wrong times of the day (and night), which I'll get into later, it's a recipe for disaster.

As I eluded to earlier, considering few companies provide their shift workers with the appropriate education and training on what to eat and when, along with how to live well whilst working 24/7; it's not surprising that most shift workers are on a treadmill of poor eating and lifestyle habits which are setting them up for chronic health conditions later down the track.

While the majority of us will do the best we can with the knowledge we have, we don't know what we don't know. In other words, we can't fix what we don't know.

Just to Clarify

Before we go any further, I do want to make mention that *Too Tired to Cook* is not a cookbook but rather a book to help motivate and inspire you to look after yourself whilst working 24/7. It's designed to educate and encourage you to do whatever it takes to look after yourself while working irregular hours. And yes, I do mean whatever it takes.

Although I am a qualified nutritionist, I didn't want this book to be all recipes; that was never my intention for writing this book. I've always had a very holistic view of health, nutrition being one of them, but there are so many other factors: sleep, as you're about to find out, being the most important.

I do, however, appreciate that people reading this book probably need guidance on what and when to eat, which is why I've included a handful of recipes in the closing chapters. While I may decide to publish a cookbook later down the track, right now, my focus is to get this book out to the world first.

After working shift work for two decades, I've realised nourishing our bodies with whole foods is extremely important (particularly if you're pushing them to the extreme, like we do when working 24/7), it's not the only thing that contributes to our health and well-being.

It's definitely an essential element given we're prone to eating all the wrong foods when we work irregular hours, but it's only one piece of an incredibly complex shift work puzzle.

The Book's Format

In the following chapters, I'm going to share with you how to manage the five biggest challenges faced by those working 24/7. I purposely chose the word *manage*, as opposed to *overcoming*, because I don't believe we can ever completely overcome them, as long as we work irregular hours.

Of course, they are by no means the only struggles faced by shift workers, but to write a book (and to avoid losing you at page number 2,864), I've purposely zoomed in on what I believe to be the most important.

The first struggle looks at sleep deprivation and disruption, which is by far the biggest Achilles heel faced by anyone who works irregular hours, and forms the real driver behind our fatigue. It's followed closely with weight fluctuations and then the combination of stress, anxiety, and depression. A depleted immune system comes in at struggle number four, before I wrap things up by going down the rabbit hole and talking all things to do with relationships. This last one is super important; we can't ignore the personal sacrifices and ramifications that working irregular hours has on those around us, including those we love and cherish.

To help put things in context, I've shared some snippets from my own shift-working life, but most importantly, I include tools and strategies you can apply so that you can begin to see positive changes in your own life, as quickly as possible.

By the time you finish reading this book, I hope you have a toolkit of ideas and actions to apply to your shift-working lifestyle. Of course, I don't have all the answers, and as I don't know you personally, not everything I write will be relevant to you. So apply what is appropriate to your situation now, and be aware of the others, because you never know when you might need to refer back to them again.

You'll also notice that I've included lots of quotes scattered throughout the pages, and at times, mentioned things more than once. That's done purely to help drive home my message in a more concise and memorable way.

Finally, to make things easier for you, I've summarised the tools and strategies into three specific "Healthy Shift Worker Action Steps" featured at the end of each chapter. They are by no means the only tips I would recommend, but again, to keep this book reasonably short, I capped them to three per struggle. So with five struggles, that's fifteen things that are going to make a massive difference in improving the quality of your life while working 24/7 (if, of course, you put them into action).

Which raises an important point: After reading this book, what are you going to do with this information? Because acquiring knowledge makes you smarter, but it certainly doesn't make you healthier.

> *Acquiring knowledge makes you smarter, but it doesn't make you healthier. That requires action.*

That requires action.

So thank you for purchasing this book, for putting your faith and trust in me to help you to manage one of the most challenging work environments in the world today.

Although I may not know you personally, please know that I genuinely do care, and I want to help transform your shift-working life into a much healthier one.

So let's begin our journey together by discussing one of the biggest struggles every shift worker experiences: sleep deprivation and disruption. This disruption to our natural sleep/wake cycle (or circadian rhythms), being the leading contributor to our ongoing fatigue.

Part 3.
The Struggles Are Real, and How to Manage Them

Struggle 1: Ongoing and Relentless Sleep Deprivation and Disruption

---

There is that level of tiredness
where you don't actually even notice you're tired,
because you no longer remember how not being tired feels.
—Arianna Huffington

Da, da, da, da! Da, da, da, da!

"Argh."

Da, da, da, da! Da, da, da, da!

"Hmmm."

Da, da, da, da! Da, da, da, da!

"Seriously, what is that noise?"

As I turned over and leaned towards my bedside table, where my alarm clock sat proudly belting out that most inhospitable sound, I opened my eyes and read the numbers: 0145.

It can't be.

As I struggled to focus my eyes, I read it again.

0145.

Surely I must be dreaming.

Alas, I was wrong.

As much as I whine and complain about my alarm clock, the one thing it doesn't do is lie. Rarely does my alarm clock get it wrong (unless, of course, the owner has programmed it incorrectly).

The reason for that inhospitable wake-up call at 0145 was because my shift at the international airport that morning was due to start at 3 a.m. (or, as we say in the aviation world, 0300), so it really was time to get up and get ready for work.

As I reluctantly dragged my body out of bed and struggled to find my balance, I staggered into the bathroom in complete darkness.

Despite being a spring chicken at the time (a mere thirtysomething years of age), every part of my body ached from top to toe.

It was after all my fifth early shift in a row, but it felt more like my tenth.

As I closed my eyes and reached across with my left hand to flick the light switch on, I grimaced. The sting of the light piercing our eyes is something we never get used to, no matter how many years we work 24/7.

I stared into the mirror at the tired and somewhat disheveled-looking image glaring back at me and said to myself, "What on earth am I doing? Can I really keep working these crazy and irregular hours?"

The bedraggled-looking image stared back at me and said nothing.

Welcome to Struggle 1, hands down the biggest challenge encountered by anyone working 24/7, that being ongoing and relentless sleep deprivation and disruption, and the subsequent fatigue associated with it.

Tired and Wired

"Everything is more difficult when you are exhausted".
—Dr Libby Weaver

If you're a shift worker reading this book right now, I'm sure you can relate to that story, or one very similar. I'm also pretty confident you've reached a point where you can't remember the last time you didn't feel tired. Except maybe when you were on holidays, and your body was finally able to catch up on some very overdue sleep.

Unfortunately, ongoing sleep deprivation and disruption come with the territory when working 24/7. It's something we inadvertently sign ourselves up for when we agree to take on the role as a shift worker, whatever that chosen occupation may be.

> *Ongoing sleep deprivation and disruption is something we inadvertently sign up for as a shift worker.*

However, lack of sleep affects every aspect of our biology, from our immune system to our digestive system to our cognitive function and even our ability to cope with stress [1]. This leaves shift workers vulnerable because sleep disruption forms such a massive part of our life. In fact, it is our life.

How Much Sleep Are We Actually Getting (or Not Getting)?

According to the Victorian State Government, shift workers get on average two to three hours less sleep than other workers, which is massive, so it's no wonder we feel exhausted [2]. When we multiply those figures per week, per month, and then per year, we end up accumulating a sleep debt we essentially can never pay back.

So despite the research saying people spend one-third of their lives sleeping [3], I'm going to add a little disclaimer to that statement and say, "Except, of course, if you're a shift worker!"

Interestingly, as luck would have it, as I write this book, the Australian Government just launched a world-first inquiry into sleep health awareness in Australia, which can I say makes me extraordinarily happy. According to the document published by the House of Representatives Standing Committee on Health, Aged Care and Sport in April 2019 [4], the committee recommended the following:

> *The development of a nationally consistent approach to working hours and rest breaks for shift workers and guidelines on how organisations should optimise rosters to minimise the potential for disruption to employee's sleep patterns.*

To say this is a positive and exciting development for those living in Australia is a massive understatement. I look forward to seeing these recommendations being put into practice, and am hopeful this initiative will set a precedent for other countries around the world to follow suit, so watch this space.

What Is Sleep, and Why Do We Need It?

"We may be what we eat, but also, to be sure, we are how we sleep."
—Arianna Huffington

Sleep. It's so incredibly elusive when working 24/7, yet imperative to our survival. Not only does it allow our body to rest, but it affects pretty much every type of cell, tissue, and system in the body, from the brain, heart, and lungs to metabolism, immune function, mood, and, most notably, the resistance of disease [5].

Unfortunately, thanks to a few early shifts or night shifts, our sleep tank is usually running on empty. Not only is the quantity of our sleep reduced when we work shift work, but so too is our sleep architecture or sleep cycles, which can compound the effects even more [6].

> *Not only is the quantity of our sleep reduced when we work shift work, but so too are our sleep cycles.*

The actual process of sleep involves passing through various cycles, each lasting around ninety to one hundred twenty minutes. They include being awake, transitioning from being awake to sleep (stage 1), light sleep (stage 2), deep or slow-wave sleep (stages 3 and 4), and rapid eye movement (REM) sleep [7]. However, when we disrupt these sleep cycles, which is often the case when working 24/7, we're going to feel the effects of sleep deprivation even more than if we were running on limited hours of sleep alone.

In other words, it's not all about the quantity of our sleep. Sleep quality is just as important, if not more, in the context of better sleep.

Two biological systems primarily regulate our sleep: the sleep/wake homeostasis, or sleep drive, and the circadian biological clock, or sleep rhythm.

If we have been awake for a long time, the sleep/wake homeostasis mechanism kicks in to remind us that we need to sleep. This drive to sleep is triggered by the build-up of a chemical in the brain called adenosine, so the longer we are awake, the higher the level of adenosine in our brain, which causes us to become sleepy [8][9].

In contrast, our circadian biological clock, located in the suprachiasmatic nuclei (SCN) of the hypothalamus of our brain (try saying those words quickly after a night of sleep deprivation!), is not only a mouthful to pronounce; it's considered the master gland of our body's hormonal system. It controls the timing of sleepiness and wakefulness throughout the day. In other words, the

SCN helps to coordinate various functions throughout the body, by ensuring they occur at certain times of the day or night, one of which is sleep [10].

The trouble for shift workers is that we often have to ignore these internal sleep drive and circadian clock cues and push our bodies to keep going, which is no easy feat when our brain and body are telling us to do the opposite. Hello, copious amounts of caffeine and sugar-laden doughnuts, and an expanding waistline, to boot!

Let's also put things into context on just how vital sleep is for our survival. During war time, sleep deprivation was (and still is) used as a form of torture [11]. So if you've ever had those moments when going into work feels like torture, you've now got a legitimate reason as to why, in more ways than one!

This highlights an important point. While air and water may surpass our fundamental need for sleep, sleep is actually more important than the food we eat.

I know what you're thinking: *Audra, you're a nutritionist. Surely you've got that wrong?*

Well, you're right. I'm definitely an advocate for eating wholesome and nutritious food. But I'm going to set the cat amongst the pigeons, so to speak (or should that be the "pillow amongst the Greek salad"?) and declare that sleep is even more important than food.

What?

Yup. Let me explain.

If you didn't eat for seven days (which I'm not recommending, by the way, as some new fancy diet for 2019), you'd undoubtedly feel weak, hungry, and a few kilograms lighter. But if you went without sleep for a week (or even just for a few days), you'd barely be able to function and begin to hallucinate [12].

Plus, and this is super-duper relevant for shift workers, our mitochondria, which are the tiny organelles located in every cell of our body that are responsible for providing us with energy, are unable to repair and regenerate if our body hasn't been able to obtain sufficient deep and restful sleep.

What exactly does that mean?

It means that you're going to be forever tired, no matter how good your nutritional and dietary intake, if you don't allow your body to sleep.

Even Professor Matthew Walker, a neuroscientist and author of the compelling book *Why We Sleep*, has stated sleep's importance over nutrition and exercise, but if you still don't believe me, please go and pick

> *You're going to be forever tired no matter how good your nutritional intake, if you don't allow your body to sleep.*

up his book and read it from cover to cover. Trust me, your views and opinions on sleep will never be the same again [13].

Brainwashing: The Kind that You Do Want to Get while Sleeping

Not only does sleep help the body to rest and repair, but it's also during this time the brain can remove toxins which have built up throughout the day, as a result of being awake. What's quite profound about this process is that the brain can only remove these toxins when we're sleeping, so lack of sleep literally prevents the clearance of toxic substances from the brain [14]. Not a particularly pleasant thought, but just something to ponder the next time you agree to do a double shift.

One of these toxins includes a protein fragment called beta-amyloid, which is strongly associated with the development of Alzheimer's disease [15]. Now I'm by no means saying that shift work leads to Alzheimer's disease. I'm merely pointing out that a lack of sleep can (and does) impair cognitive function in many ways, and there's plenty of research confirming this. One study involving more than a thousand shift workers, and published in the *Journal of Occupational and Environmental Medicine*, identified an association between impaired cognition in subjects who had worked shift work for more than ten years [16].

Now I know what you're thinking: It's not the rosiest of news, but it's crucial that you're aware of it, particularly when I run through some of the tips and strategies on how to improve the quality and quantity of your sleep, especially tip number 1. I also don't want any long-term shift workers reading this to panic because there is good news. Recovery from cognitive decline can occur; however, according to this particular study, it can take at least five years after leaving shift work. It's why a big focus of this book is going to be around protecting your sleep because sleep is sacred, and we need to be treating it as such.

So how exactly does this brainwashing work when we're sleeping? Well, unlike the lymphatic system, which is like an internal plumbing system that removes wastes and toxins from our body 24/7, there is no lymph in our brain. Instead, there is something called the *glymphatic* system, which is the brain's own waste disposal system and functions in a similar way to the lymphatic system. During sleep, the glymphatic system becomes ten times more active, and the cells of our brain shrink in size by approximately 60 percent, providing space so that the cerebral spinal fluid can wash and remove the toxins from the brain more effectively [17].

Pretty phenomenal? So never underestimate the importance of sleep and assume that you can run on four to five hours a night, day after day, night after night, year after year, and it not affect your cognition, amongst other things. The results may not be noticeable straight away, but it's highly likely that it will rear its ugly head in years to come, just as it did for me, ten years into my shift-working career, and at the tender age of thirtysomething.

Case Study 1. Forgetting the Names of My Workmates

I was walking down the concourse at the domestic airport one day and passed one of my colleagues, who was walking in the other direction.

"Hi, Audra, how are you going?"

"Hi [oh, my gosh; I've forgotten her name]. I'm good, thanks. How are you?"

Thankfully, she didn't appear too worried that I hadn't replied using her name.

Phew.

I was only thirty-six years old, a little young to be experiencing dementia.

Or was I?

Interestingly enough, I did begin to notice the decline in my memory in my early thirties, but it only became noticeable when I started to forget the names of people I worked with, people I'd worked with and known for years, but somehow, I'd forget their name.

How could this happen? Was I losing my mind? Because this didn't just happen once or twice; it became a regular occurrence.

I would often try and hide it by pretending to make a joke about the situation. If someone greeted me with a "Hi, Audra," and I couldn't remember his name, I'd reply with a "Hi, George," knowing it wasn't right, and then follow up by joking, "Just mucking around," to try and hide my embarrassment.

In the meantime, I would go through the alphabet in my head, hoping it would trigger my memory. Sometimes it worked; sometimes it didn't. Either way, I sensed the effects of sleep deprivation must have been a contributing factor in the decline in my cognitive function, but like many shift workers, I just accepted that it is what it is and got on with it.

Ironically, it wasn't until I went back to university and began to delve into some of the science behind the cumulative effects of ongoing sleep deprivation that my inability to remember my workmate's names became so much clearer.

How to Improve Your Sleep

We know shift workers experience sleep deprivation and disruption, thanks to our haphazard schedules, but what can we do to improve the situation? Well, before I flood you with some ninja sleep-enhancing strategies, I'd like to point out that this book will list many healthy shift-worker strategies, with the most important strategy first. This is because I want to cut to the chase and help you to feel better in the fastest time possible.

These strategies will incorporate things we can change, as opposed to those we have no control over, because when we focus on the latter, it adds to our futility and can deplete our energy even more. For example, we may not be able to change our roster and sleep as well as our 9–5 non-shift-working cousins, who have the luxury of a regular routine (believe me, I'd love to be able to wave a magic wand over your schedules to make them more user-friendly). I have to be realistic in my approach.

So hold on to your hats (or should I say pillows?) and get ready to receive some sleep-induced inspiration as I share my top three sleep essentials to help with sleep deprivation and disruption; it can be ongoing and relentless, but these tips will help you reclaim some of that energy that got up and vanished since you began working 24/7.

1. Prioritise Your Sleep, No Matter What

> *"The number of people who can survive on six hours sleep*
> *without showing any impairment … is zero."*
> —Professor Matthew Walker

You may be thinking, *Of all the things you could suggest for a shift worker, Audra, that's what you've come up with? That's your number one recommendation?* Well, before you're tempted to throw this book at me (thankfully, that's not possible), stick with me here because while prioritising our sleep might sound obvious, especially when we're running on a deficit, many of us fail to do so, even when working 24/7. Some people even brag about how *little* sleep they are getting. If you know of anyone like that, please give them a copy of this book.

> *Prioritizing our sleep might sound obvious, yet so many of us fail to do so, even when working 24/7.*

You can also take all the prescription medications and supplements that you want, or eat the best diet in the world, but if you do not focus on prioritising your sleep, then it's like driving around through life with the handbrake on.

So if there's one key takeaway that you get from reading this book, it's making sleep your number 1 priority, period.

Because when we combine a disrupted circadian rhythm with poor sleep habits, it's going to accelerate your brain fog and fatigue, and lead to a whole host of other health complaints.

Of course, I'm sure you can relate to partying into the wee hours of the morning at some point in time, despite having an early shift the next day. Or gone straight from a night shift to attend your child's school music recital on little to no sleep. I get it. We've all done it, but if this is a regular occurrence, please don't fool yourself. You need more sleep.

As Matthew Walker so eloquently states in *Why We Sleep*, "The number of people who can survive on 6 hours sleep without showing any impairment, rounded to a whole number and expressed as a percentage of the population, is zero."

Whilst we can certainly bounce back after a night of sleep deprivation much better when we're in our twenties, as opposed to our forties and fifties or sixties, how we take care of ourselves now will definitely have an impact on our health later in life.

Let's take our obsession with staying up late and spending countless hours on our electronic devices, along with staring aimlessly into the glowing screens of our flat-screened TVs. While I'll go into more detail on this in tip number two, this sleep-sabotaging behaviour cuts into our already very depleted, running-on-empty sleep status. Today's fixation with our phones has been touted as an addiction on par with tobacco and alcohol [18]. There's even a name for it: it's called *nomophobia*, as in fear of no-mo(bile) phone, and it affects up to 40 percent of the population [19]. I'd hazard a guess that it is much higher right now, considering this research was published back in 2013.

It's also highly likely that our lack of priority for sleep coincides with our current world of busyness, as in that all-too-common response we hear from so many people these days: "I'm just so busy." However, sacrificing our sleep to get things done is not a good habit to get into, particularly when the sleep tank is already sitting dangerously in the red zone.

I remember when one of my lovely clients said to me, "I've kind of put sleep on the back burner. I've got too many other things to do than sleep."

The thing is, many of us think we can get more done if we sleep less, but in reality, our productivity takes a nosedive, and we're more likely to make mistakes when we don't get sufficient sleep [20].

What's even more frightening is that after eighteen hours without sleep, our performance is worse than if we had a blood alcohol reading of 0.05 percent [21]. Yes, you read that correctly. You are effectively drunk after eighteen hours without sleep.

So the next time you choose to work a double shift and then get into your car to drive home, please remember that your cognitive function and reaction times are going to be impaired like someone legally drunk, but without drinking a single drop of

> *The next time you decide to do a double shift and get into the car to drive home, remember that your cognition and reaction times are going to be impaired as if you were legally drunk.*

alcohol. I'm sure I don't need to point out that the ramifications of this decision can be disastrous, not only for you but for others on the road.

Now don't get me wrong. I know that sometimes, for whatever reason, we may be required to work a double or longer than usual shift, but it certainly should not be the norm. I also get that people are busy. Juggling shift work with everyday life, including running a household, raising kids, and study commitments, is a pretty big ask, but despite what you may think, you're not superhuman.

You *need* sleep, and those around you (most notably your loved ones), need you to get sufficient amounts of sleep too.

2. Boot Your Phone out of the Bedroom

Okay. So I think now is the time to bring up a somewhat-sensitive topic, that being not only who you're inviting into your bedroom (which, by the way, is entirely up to you!) but what you're bringing into your bedroom. I think we can all agree, many of our bedrooms these days are looking more like a bed-office, than a bed-room.

In fact, in the last ten years, we've morphed into a new species, one that's gained an extra appendage of sorts, which is distracting us to the point that we're no longer talking to each other.

This extra appendage, of course, being our mobile phones.

While these trusty little gadgets are amazing at what they can do (from taking a photo to delivering food to our doorstep), they're also great at taking away precious minutes, hours, and weeks from our everyday lives, including that all-important opportunity to sleep.

You might think, *Weeks? That's a bit of an exaggeration, isn't it, Audra?*

Trust me; I'm not making this up. When we begin to track precisely how much time we're spending on our phones, minutes turn into hours, hours turn into weeks, weeks turn into … well, you get my drift.

Quite simply, we're severely underestimating exactly how much time we're spending on our phones.

And the one thing about time is that we can never get it back.

Once it's gone, it's gone forever.

> *She was quite simply giving away an hour and a half of precious sleep time that she would never get back.*

I remember one of my clients saying that she would go to bed around nine o'clock but would be straight on her phone to watch Netflix, along with scrolling through Facebook or Instagram, chatting with her girlfriends. Before she knew it, it would be eleven o'clock. She was quite simply giving away an hour and a half of precious sleep time that she would never get back. Not to mention, this constant exposure to information is beyond the comprehension of our ancestors, and it's having negative consequences on our health [22].

So when I suggested to her to go on a mobile phone and social media 'fast' to help with her sleep, her response to me was "Wow – heaven! I can't wait!" Given our addiction to social media and our mobile phones these days I nearly fell of my chair because it's definitely not the usual response that I get from my clients. Suffice to say I was very

ⸯ hear it, and even more happy to hear that her sleep improved
ⸯsly as a result of implementing this strategy.

ⸯthing is, we need to give ourselves sufficient opportunity to
sleep because it's a process. It doesn't happen instantly. Our body
needs time to wind down. So please, if this self-sabotaging sleep
behaviour of scrolling through your phone mindlessly before bed is
something you do, I urge you to start tracking your mobile phone use
so that you can become aware of just how much time you're spending
on your phone. By correcting this self-sabotaging habit, you can
regain some of that precious sleep your body so desperately needs.

Light and Stimulation Are Not Your Friends

Not only are our mobile phones becoming time zappers, but the
blue light emitting from electronic devices such as phones, laptops,
and iPads also disrupts our ability to fall asleep and stay asleep. They
disrupt our sleep/wake cycle, or circadian rhythms, as much as the
shift work itself.

These blue screens (technically, it's considered a white light)
disrupt our delicate endocrine system by suppressing the release
of a vital sleep-regulating hormone called melatonin. At the same
time, it's activating arousal-promoting orexin neurons, along with
stimulating the "fight-or-flight" arm of our nervous system, which is
involved in the stress response [23] [24] [25]

This is not good, as stress and sleep do not mix well together.

Of course, a lot of us are guilty of using television, computers,
smartphones, and tablets as a way of winding down and relaxing after
work. However, this obsession with electronic devices is not doing us
any favours when it comes to topping up the sleep tank. Quite simply,
the light changes our biochemistry, which has a flow-on effect on
our sleep.

It's why we're currently seeing an influx of blue-light blocking glasses coming onto the market, as they help to reduce some effects of light toxicity, along with helping to protect our mitochondria. Mitochondria are those tiny organelles located within our cells that convert nutrients from the food that we eat into energy. Ahh, energy. Do you remember what that is? It's a state of being that seems to magically disappear when we commence working 24/7, as I'm sure you can relate.

While I am a big fan of wearing these light-blocking glasses 1 hour before bed to help protect our eyes and mitochondria, along with stimulating melatonin production, we need to ensure we're implementing the common-sense practices first. That is booting our phone out of the bedroom and replacing it with a good old-fashioned alarm clock.

"But, Audra, I use my mobile phone as an alarm clock!"

Ahh yes, a response I hear often. Believe it or not, there are such things as alarm clocks. These fantastic devices come in all different shapes, colours, and sizes, and are highly trained in the art of waking you up, as opposed to distracting you when you should be sleeping.

Pretty incredible, hey?

So my challenge to you right now, starting from tonight, is to boot your mobile phone out of your bedroom, and if you don't already have one, buy yourself a good old-fashioned alarm clock, one that's not going to jolt you into consciousness like an electric shock but, instead, wake you more gently because your nervous system is already tired, wired, and on-edge as a result of ongoing sleep disruption.

Now there are plenty of super fancy alarm clocks on the market right now, including ones that once you hit the snooze button, start to move away from you, creating enough distance that you have to get out of bed to turn it off. I chuckle at the thought of trying to turn one of those off, in the pitch-black darkness, at 3 a.m! There are even alarm clocks that simulate a sunrise, but this is probably not ideal if you're sharing your bed with someone who doesn't have to get up at crazy o'clock with you [26].

I'm all about keeping things simple. Just head on down to your local K-Mart or Target and search for the most basic alarm clock you can find that emits minimal (if any) light. I'm not exaggerating by telling you this will be an absolute game-changer. I've seen it time and time again with my clients. Their results have been nothing short of life-changing when it comes to improving their sleep.

3. Focus on Relaxation, Not Sedation

One of the biggest misconceptions when it comes to why shift workers struggle to fall asleep and stay asleep is that we're not going to bed relaxed. This could be due to a myriad of reasons, but many shift workers experience difficulty switching off or winding down especially after a busy shift.

> *In order to sleep, and sleep well, we must be relaxed.*

The thing is, in order to sleep, and sleep well, we must be relaxed, but so many of us are making matters worse by not allowing our body to transition into a place of calm. Prioritising our sleep and booting the phone out of the bedroom is the very first step towards reclaiming that relaxation status.

Despite our strong desire to want to fall asleep quickly, particularly when we've got one of those nasty quick-turnaround shifts, sleep cannot be magically turned on and off as quickly and easily as a light switch. Especially if our bodies are not relaxed.

It's not that simple.

Of course, there are those times when we're so exhausted that as soon as our head hits the pillow, we're out like a light, but for many, those times are few and far between.

It's why many shift workers resort to popping a pill, with the expectation of being able to fall asleep and stay asleep, with little effort. However, this popping-a-pill-to-fall-asleep strategy, especially when it comes to using pharmaceutical medications such as benzodiazepines and Z-drugs, can be a dangerous path to follow. This is because these man-made, synthetic medications can be addictive and often come with nasty side effects, not to mention they're not designed for long-term use, despite people taking them for months and even years at a time [27].

One of the best books written on the subject of pharmaceutical sleep medications is *Undrugged: Sleep from Insomnia to Un-somnia: Why Sleeping Pills Don't Improve Sleep and the Drug-Free Solutions That Will*. It's a real eye-opener on the world of sleep medications and written by pharmacist Dr Lori Arnold, who is more than qualified to talk all things pharmaceuticals.

As Dr Arnold so eloquently states in her book, we need to acknowledge that taking a pill is not addressing the root cause as to why you're experiencing insomnia (besides the shift work itself); there could be other factors contributing to your inability to fall asleep and stay asleep that are not being addressed.

Personally, and this is purely my opinion, but when you look at how these sleep medications work, it doesn't make sense for shift workers to take them. This is because many have a sedative or hypnotic effect.

Now correct me if I'm wrong, but shift workers don't need to be sedated or hypnotised. We're already walking around as though we're in some kind of drug-

> *Shift workers don't need to be sedated or hypnotised. We're already walking around as though we're in some kind of drug-induced state, thanks to a disruptive sleep lifestyle.*

induced state, as we struggle to string two words together, along with trying to ascertain what day of the week it is or whether we've fed the cat (or even the kids)!

We also need to appreciate that a drug-induced sleep is not real sleep. It doesn't offer the same restorative and reparative qualities as a true night's sleep, which is why we need to help our body relax and transition into sleep on its own, as much as we possibly can [28].

Which all comes back to relaxation and having more of a holistic lifestyle approach, as opposed to a "Let's take a pill to knock me out" approach.

But there's a catch.

It takes work.

It takes effort and a commitment on your part to get yourself feeling relaxed, so that you, in turn, can fall asleep. Quite simply, you must be willing to put in the effort, put yourself first, and implement self-care strategies consistently, no matter what.

Yes, this even applies if you're a parent who is juggling a job around children or taking care of elderly parents or some other commitment. If anything, you need to make a pact to implement self-care even more, so that your body gets the opportunity to relax and sleep, instead of running on adrenalin and being on the brink of burnout.

Self-Care 101

So if you're struggling to fall asleep or stay asleep, it's time to get serious. It's time to give your sleep-sabotaging behaviours an honest review and replace them with some self-care strategies to shift your body into relaxation mode, as opposed to knocking yourself out with a sedative.

Now don't get me wrong. I'm not here to judge anyone. If you're taking sleep medications, and you've found them to be helpful, that's fantastic.

I mean that sincerely.

I put my hand on my heart when I say I want shift workers everywhere to get better quality sleep. All I ask is that you make sure you're well aware of the risks versus benefits of being on these medications, particularly long-term.

Your sleep quality is going to be so much better, and you'll wake up feeling a zillion times better if you're able to help your body to transition into sleep more naturally. This is our body's innate intelligence.

Now, of course, everybody relaxes differently, but to sleep, and sleep well, you need to give your body the chance to move into what's called parasympathetic mode, which is just a fancy way to describe the rest-and-digest arm of the nervous system.

You can't be in fight-or-flight stress mode and rest-and-digest mode at the same time, if you want to get better sleep.

Sorry to burst your bubble, but it just isn't going to happen!

So it's up to you whether you incorporate the use of blue-light blocking glasses, essential oils, sound therapy, yoga, meditation, or mindfulness strategies which, by the way, are not some hippy-type strategies that don't work. Ask anyone who uses these practices regularly (*regular* being the keyword), and you'll be amazed at how well they do work.

One of my favourite ways of relaxing is using diaphragmatic breathing, also referred to as abdominal breathing or belly breathing. According to the Harvard Medical School, diaphragmatic breathing helps to slow the heart rate down, decrease blood pressure, and improve sleep: a winning combination for anyone working 24/7 [29]. It also has a powerful anti-anxiety effect, which is essential given many people struggle to sleep because they're unable to switch off their racing mind or suffer from anxiety (even around not being able to sleep).

There are a few different versions, but one in particular, known as the "4-7-8 breathing technique" involves breathing in for 4 counts, holding for 7, and then breathing out for 8; one of the best things about this practice is that it's extremely time efficient, in that it only takes a minute or two to do. Most importantly, when done consistently, it can have dramatic improvements not only on your sleep but on your overall health and well-being too.

For instructions on how to implement diaphragmatic breathing, check out Dr Andrew Weil's YouTube video titled "Asleep in 60 Seconds: 4-7-8 Breathing Technique Claims to Help You to Nod off in Just a Minute." It will feel strange at first, and probably take a few goes to get used to it, but if you stick with it, it has the potential to be life-changing when it comes to improving your sleep [30].

If you're feeling doubtful that something so simple could actually improve your sleep, then you might want to read this testimonial from a lady who attended one of my Healthy Shift Worker Workplace Wellness events, and then sent me this message about a week later.

Case Study 2. *Sue's Post-Night-Shift Success Story

"I have always slept well as a shift worker but was intrigued by your breathing technique for inducing sleep. I have just finished night shift and am over the moon to say that I averaged 9 hours sleep each day, thanks to the breathe in for 4, hold 567, and exhale on 8. I used this every morning to get to sleep and only remember doing it three or four times before I was out like a light.

I've spread the word to all who would listen (and some who didn't care). What a wonderful technique. Thank you for improving my quality of sleep on night shift."

---

*For privacy reasons, this is not her real name

Just One More Thing: Are You Eating to Relax?

"When your diet is full of stimulants like caffeine and refined sugar, and <u>devoid of nutrients</u>, your body cannot make the necessary hormones for calm, and to create your sleep hormones."
—Dr Libby Weaver

As a nutritionist, I couldn't end this chapter without mentioning the importance of nutrition when it comes to our sleep, because what we eat can have a profound impact on our ability (or inability) to sleep.

This was highlighted in a study published in the *Journal of Clinical Sleep Medicine* where eating less fibre, more saturated fat, and more sugar was associated with lighter, less restorative, and more disrupted sleep [31].

I hate to say it, but that sounds like the typical shift worker's diet right there.

Other studies have shown how high-fat diets can lead to daytime sleepiness and poor sleep [32], while an animal study published in *Cell Metabolism* identified that overeating, along with consuming a diet high in processed fats, can disrupt our body clock [33]. As if our body clocks aren't disrupted enough just from working 24/7!

Even excess salt consumption before bed can affect sleep quality by increasing sleep disturbances, reducing deep sleep, and triggering the need to get up and drink water [34]. So munching on that packet of salty crisps, nuts, or fries before bed may not be a great idea if you want to move into relaxation mode and wake up feeling refreshed.

Okay, I think the term *semi-refreshed* is more appropriate for anyone working 24/7, but the point I'm trying to get across is that if your diet is made up predominantly of processed and refined foods, then it's highly likely that it's impacting on your ability to relax and sleep well.

Healthy Shift Worker Action Steps

1. Prioritise your sleep, no matter what.
2. Boot your phone out of the bedroom.
3. Focus on relaxation, not sedation.

Struggle 2: My Uniform Must Be Shrinking - Weight Fluctuations and an Expanding Waistline

---

"We are not only what we eat, but when we eat."
—Franz Halberg

It was a cold, chilly winter's day as I jumped out of the shower and began getting dressed for a late shift that afternoon, when all of a sudden, I heard a noise.

Pop! Ping, ping, ping.

"What the?"

As I turned my head and glanced around the room to see where this unusual sound came from, I looked down and noticed a button missing off the jacket of my uniform.

That's odd, I thought. *I wonder what happened to my missing button?*

To my disbelief, I soon realised that weird pinging noise was one of my buttons shearing off my jacket and ricocheting off the wall, before eventually coming to rest in the bottom of my empty bathtub.

I looked down at my uniform to where my missing button once lived, and all I could see were a few strands of thread.

As I made a second attempt to secure my jacket, I soon realised that no matter how hard I stretched that uniform, the missing button and buttonhole were never going to meet and come together as one.

"How could that be?" I asked myself.

Had my uniform shrunk? Did the dry cleaners inadvertently shrink my jacket?

That must be it. I mean, something untoward must have happened to my uniform causing it to shrink in size.

That was the only explanation possible.

Or was it?

As I stood before the mirror, looking at the half-dressed image, something didn't seem quite right. Either the jacket had indeed shrunk, or the contents within that jacket had outgrown its size.

The contents, of course, being me.

But how could that be possible?

Had I outgrown my uniform? Had my jacket become a casualty of my expanding waistline?

Hard to comprehend, given I'd always been fairly skinny. My sister often called me "Emu Legs" as a result of my long and lanky limbs (sisters: You've got to love them).

But the reality was, I'd never had a weight problem, ever.

I was always the skinny, long-legged kid who could pretty much eat anything and never put on any weight.

Until now.

It was at that moment that I came to the realisation that my sedentary lifestyle, irregular eating schedule, and poor food choices had finally caught up with me at the tender age of twenty-four.

The endless packets of chips, two-minute noodles, blocks of chocolate, diet soft drinks, and all the other questionable food that had become a part of my daily intake had eventually led to an unprecedented amount of pressure on the seams of my uniform, to a point where the button could no longer hold those bits of fabric together.

So while I wanted to blame a shrinking uniform for the fate of my jacket that day, the harsh reality was that my actions leading up to that point had become a significant contributor to my weight gain. And even though I only gained around fifteen

> *My actions had become a major contributor to my weight gain, something I chose to ignore for many years, before finally accepting responsibility and doing something about it.*

kilograms, it felt like a lot more on my long and lanky frame.

When I look back now, having since graduated as a nutritionist and having a much better understanding of how my body works, the weight gain wasn't the real concern. Of real concern was that my body had become quite puffy, particularly around my face and hands, which is a sign of inflammation, one of the leading causes of many chronic health conditions.

Incredibly, despite the discomfort of the added weight, I pretty much chose to ignore it for many years, before finally accepting responsibility and doing something about it.

The catalyst for that change was when I stumbled across a book by Cyndi O'Meara called *Changing Habits, Changing Lives*, and the rest, as they say, is history.

Sounding Familiar?

I think everyone who has ever worked shift work before can relate to this or a similar story, at some point in their career. Weight fluctuations and shift work are quite synonymous with one another, which is why an expanding waistline is next on my hit list of some of the biggest struggles of working 24/7.

But why is this so? Why is it that as a result of working 24/7, the seams of our clothes become stretched to a point where they break and unravel in a chaotic mess?

The answer to this question can be quite complex, but as shift workers, we are often plagued by constant fatigue and tiredness with little energy to cook; so before we know it, we're heading down a path of poor eating habits, coupled with a sedentary lifestyle. In other words, ongoing sleep deprivation can lead to changes in our behaviour that, over time, will literally stretch the limit on the seams of our clothes.

Why Your Expanding Waistline Is Not Entirely Your Fault

Whenever we're feeling run down and tired (welcome to the wonderful world of shift work), we don't always make the healthiest food choices.

It's kind of obvious, but why is that?

Why is it that whenever we're running on little sleep, we're magnetically drawn to the sugar-laden candy bars from the vending machine or the greasy chips and gravy from the workplace cafeteria?

Well, it could be due to many reasons, and not just lack of willpower.

One of these includes the effect sleep deprivation has on our brain. Studies have shown sleep deprivation impairs the frontal lobe region of the brain which is involved in making complex decisions, while simultaneously, increasing activity in the deeper area of the brain called the amygdala, which is involved in reward-seeking behaviour [1].

In other words, our tired brains are more geared to eating for pleasure, as opposed to hunger, so we're more likely to crave and seek out the sweet and fatty foods which are not ideal, given carbohydrate metabolism becomes impaired during sleep loss [23].

So there you go, you now have a valid reason for craving the pizza, doughnuts, happy meals, and fries while working 24/7.

Please note that I used the word "reason", and not justification!

To add to our woes, portion sizes tend to increase when we're running on little sleep [4], with one particular study showing substantial increases in weight and caloric consumption of up to an additional 550 calories per day [5]. This may be due to an elevation in the stress hormone cortisol due to chronic stress associated with a lack of sleep, which increases our appetite and redistributes fat stores around our waist [6].

You're probably thinking, there goes any chance of reacquainting yourself with that svelte figure that you had as a teenager!

Well, for most people that's going to be a big ask anyway, so if this is you, you may be putting a lot of unnecessary pressure on yourself. At the same time, we shouldn't be adopting the "I'm just getting older" mentality either, because that can make us complacent when it comes to taking care of our health.

It's Not All about the Number

It's incredible how many of us measure our self-worth by a number on a bathroom scale. While I'm not saying that we shouldn't be paying attention to it, it's the *location* of the weight or, more specifically, the distribution of the body fat that we need to be keeping a watchful eye on. This is because, when we have high amounts of fat deposited around the belly (otherwise known as central adiposity), it puts pressure on the organs as well as raising our risk for developing conditions such as heart disease, diabetes, and even premature death [6]. Excess weight and body fat also increase our likelihood of developing obstructive sleep apnea, which is not great for shift workers as this intensifies the effects of sleep loss even further [7].

Another reason your weight gain may not be entirely your fault is that sleep deprivation alters our appetite-regulating hormones ghrelin and leptin, which can cause havoc on our appetite and, over time, our waistline [8]. Leptin is a hormone that tells us when we're feeling full, and ghrelin is a hormone that tells us when we're hungry. I like to refer to ghrelin as the "tummy growl hormone" as it sends messages to our brain telling us that we're hungry.

But here's the trap for anyone working 24/7 …

When we're tired, our body increases production of this "tummy growl hormone," while at the same time, reducing leptin. In other words, thanks to our sleep-deprived lifestyle, we're going to experience higher rates of appetite and hunger than if we'd had plenty of sleep. It also makes us more prone to over-eating as leptin; the "I'm feeling full" hormone becomes suppressed on limited amounts of sleep [8]. This was illustrated in a study where people who slept only four hours for two nights in a row, experienced an 18 percent reduction in leptin, and a 28 percent increase in ghrelin [9]. It's why the only diet I will ever advocate for shift workers (because I dislike the word *diet*) is the "Sleep More Diet!"

> *The only diet I will ever advocate for shift workers is the "Sleep More Diet."*

Lastly, we must also appreciate that sleep deprivation is a form of stress which causes havoc on our stress-regulating adrenal glands, which can have a flow-on effect to our thyroid gland and metabolism. In other words, adrenal or thyroid dysfunction, or a combination of the two, can lead to a sluggish metabolism, and an ongoing struggle to lose weight [10].

How to Shrink Our Expanding Waistlines

While there is undoubtedly a lot of science and research highlighting how shift workers are prone to gaining weight, I do not believe it has to be this way. I'm a big believer in preventative medicine, which begins by gaining a better understanding of how our body works while working 24/7. Combine this with taking responsibility for our food intake and other lifestyle choices; this can go a long way in preventing ourselves from becoming another weight gain statistic.

We also can't blame shift work entirely for our weight gain, nor should we believe that we're destined to become overweight if we work 24/7.

We can't blame shift work entirely for our weight gain, nor should we believe that we're destined to become overweight if we work 24/7.

If this were true, then every single person who works shift work would be overweight, and this is not the case.

Now, before I get into the nuts and bolts of how and what to do, I don't want to come across all harsh, but if you've been steadily gaining weight over the years, then it may be time for a bit of a reality check.

As Dr Libby Weaver describes in her book, *Accidentally Overweight*, the weight gain doesn't magically appear overnight, all by itself [11].

Unlike our ancestors before us, we've become increasingly sedentary, and food has become so readily available to us; we don't even have to go out and 'hunt and gather' for it anymore.

If we choose to, we don't even have to get out of the car to find food. We drive down a little laneway, make a choice from a bulletin board, speak into a microphone, press down on the accelerator, and wait by a tiny window where our food magically appears.

All in a matter of minutes and without moving from our seat.

But let's be brutally honest. If it comes through a car window, it's not going to nourish us on a cellular level, which is exactly what our bodies need.

Instead, this endless supply of palatable and easily accessible food is causing us to overeat, and overeat on all of the wrong types of food. It causes us to become bigger and bigger, and rather than try and do something about it, we conceal our expanding waistlines by wearing clothes that camouflage all those extra bumpy bits that weren't there when we were younger.

However, let's be realistic; this is not solving the problem. It's just covering it up, literally. If we're overweight (particularly around the middle), then we need to find a way to lose the weight and get ourselves feeling healthy again.

Case Study 3. How a Cosy Trip in the Flight Deck Left Me Feeling Anxious

As an employee of the airline industry, I was often lucky enough to catch a ride home in the flight deck whenever the flights were overbooked. It was an incredible opportunity and one I will always be grateful for, as I was able to experience something most people never do in their lifetime.

However, there was one particular time, after arriving back in Sydney after an extremely long flight from Alaska, when I was able to secure the jump seat back to Brisbane (an extra seat in the cockpit reserved for additional crew), which left me feeling extremely anxious.

It was a light bulb moment of sorts, which made me even more concerned about our expanding waistlines and the subsequent ill-effects that can occur from being overweight.

As I strapped myself into the jump seat and listened in earnest to the emergency evacuation drill from the First Officer, I could not help but feel a little apprehensive. While he went through the evacuation process in the unlikely event that something catastrophic happened on the flight, he directed me to the window above his right shoulder.

His instructions were clear. In the unlikely event of an emergency landing, we will be climbing through his window as a means of escape.

I said, "Sure, no problem," but what I declined to ask (despite the obvious question spinning around in my head) was how he was going to get out through that window.

You see, I'm a relatively lean and flexible person, thanks to regular walks and yoga, so I would have had no problem jumping out that window if I had to. But the First Officer, on the other hand … well, let me say that due to the circumference of his waistline, it would have delayed our escape if the aircraft did have to make an emergency landing.

And this left me feeling anxious.

While I knew I could get out that window if I had to, I felt like my life was in the hands of someone else.

His expanding waistline could have delayed my escape from a potentially life-threatening situation.

Fortunately, there was no emergency landing; we arrived safely back into my home port of Brisbane and were able to disembark as usual, through the much wider front door of the aircraft.

But that flight home was a defining moment and a flight I will never forget.

While I hope you never have to squeeze through an aircraft window, or even a car window, for that matter, if you ever did have to do something similar to save your life or someone you love, could you do it? Is your body lean enough and flexible enough to escape an emergency if you had to? Are you physically strong enough to lift something if you had to? I'll leave those questions with you to ponder.

1. Eat Minimally When Your Digestive System Is Sleeping

"While we obsess over what to eat,
we virtually ignore the crucial aspect of meal timing.
—Dr Jason Fung

If you're only going to remember one teeny tiny thing from reading this book (in addition to prioritising your sleep), please make this section be that one little bit! Because I'm about to share with you something that is rarely mentioned and discussed in most nutritional and dietary textbooks and consultations, yet its relevance and importance cannot be overestimated, particularly for anyone working 24/7.

The topic I'm referring to is meal timing; the fancier, more scientific way to describe it is chrononutrition, a term originally coined by Dr Alain Delabos back in 1986 and based around the principles of the body's biological clock. It's since become an emerging field of research in nutritional epidemiology that encompasses three dimensions of eating behaviour: timing, frequency, and regularity. Given shift workers work 24/7 and thereby have a tendency to eat 24/7, timing and meal regularity (or in the case of shift workers, irregularity) is a very pertinent topic for discussion [12] [13].

Just to put things in context, in my final year at university to become a nutritionist back in 2016, one of the questions we would often ask clients when they came in to see us was what they ate for breakfast, lunch, dinner, and everything else in between. However, as many of my clients appeared to be eating reasonably well, but were still struggling with their weight, I began to ask a different question: *when* they were eating.

Their responses opened my eyes up to a whole new world of nutrition, as it made me curious to learn how food timing can influence our ability to lose weight. It's when I first came across the term *chrononutrition*, and my interest in wanting to learn more really gained momentum.

Especially since more and more research is emerging, identifying a distinct link between food intake irregularity as a potential risk factor for chronic diseases such as metabolic syndrome, including high blood pressure, high blood sugar, excess body fat around the waist, and abnormal cholesterol levels. This syndrome increases a person's risk of heart attack and stroke, and while the exact mechanisms are unclear, studies have suggested that consuming meals irregularly affects our internal body clock, which has a flow-on effect to our metabolism [14].

The philosophy behind chrononutrition is that we restrict our food intake to a particular time of day or eat in coordination with the body's natural daily rhythms, which typically follow a twenty-four-hour cycle. This eating as close to normal times as possible is designed to reduce our risk of developing certain metabolic disorders such as insulin resistance and obesity, conditions which are becoming increasingly common in those who work 24/7 [15] [16].

Now, for people who work 9–5 and go to bed at around the same time every night and eat their meals at similar times of the day, this is pretty easy to do. But for those of us who work different shifts, we end up falling into the trap of eating at various times of the day.

The problem with this type of ad hoc eating pattern is that altering the time we eat (regardless of what we eat) can significantly affect our body weight [16]. In essence, ingesting food during the night versus the day can have completely different effects on our metabolism, making shift workers more vulnerable to weight gain [17] [18]. This is because many nutritionally related metabolic processes in the body follow this natural daily rhythm, including our appetite, the digestion process, and the metabolism of fat, cholesterol, and glucose [14].

Quite simply, the human body has not evolved to eat 24/7. Just like our ancestors

> *Ingesting food during the night versus the day can have completely different effects on our metabolism, making shift workers vulnerable to weight gain.*

did before us, we're meant to endure periods of scarcity, where we don't eat. But in this day and age, we have access to food all the time, so we feel obliged to eat 24/7 [15].

However, certain organs such as the liver, pancreas, and intestine methodically follow a twenty-four-hour rhythm; they don't expect food intake at 3 a.m. So when you munch on that pizza after midnight while on the night shift, when your body is usually sound asleep in bed (and you wish that you were at home in bed too), it's going to struggle to digest it.

> Our body is not geared up for night-time energy and nutrient consumption.

Primarily, our body is not geared for night-time energy and nutrient consumption; gastric emptying, intestinal blood flow, kidney, and liver activity all slow down during the night [19]. This can be one of the reasons why we experience indigestion, pain, and discomfort when working (and eating) on the night shift.

In addition, circadian misalignment, which is just a fancy way to describe our disrupted sleep/wake cycle, can be a contributing factor in the ever-growing rise in the incidence of diabetes amongst the shift-working population because it impairs our glucose tolerance. In other words, it struggles to remove blood sugar from the cells. This is because pancreatic β-cell function, the organ and cells responsible for releasing insulin to reduce blood sugar, is reduced at night [20].

This makes reducing your intake of processed sugars and refined carbohydrates at night even more critical, not only from a weight gain perspective, but because your blood sugar levels will remain much higher than if you ate the same thing during the daytime [20].

Even animal studies have shown eating during irregular sleeping hours promotes increased body weight and accumulates abdominal fat, whereas when food is consumed by following the natural sleep/wake cycle or circadian rhythm, such weight gain wasn't seen [21].

So while *what* we eat is important, when we eat, or the time of ingestion, is just as critical (if not more so) for our well-being [22].

Of course, I'm not advising you avoid food intake altogether while on the night shift, although this does work for some people. It's more about limiting your food intake, especially during the night when your digestive system is mostly sleeping (or at least trying to), as it will do wonders for your metabolic health and waistline [15].

> *Limiting your food intake during the night will do wonders for your metabolic health and waistline.*

Foods which are more suitable to consume while working overnight are going to be those which have a minimal effect on your blood sugar and insulin levels, such as low-carbohydrate foods, along with those which require little digestive effort. For example, more plant-based protein and liquid nutrition-type meals such as soups, smoothies, along with bone broths or stocks, as they are super healing on the gut.

Reducing Your Feeding Window to Amplify Autophagy

You're probably wondering, what on earth is autophagy? Well, it's actually the body's way of cleaning out damaged cells to allow for the regeneration of newer, healthier cells. So it's kind of important.

The thing is, for most shift workers, we need to be reducing the length of time that we're eating over a 24-hour period. This is because autophagy is a process that usually occurs while we're sleeping and fasting through the night, but as shift workers, we're often awake and eating instead.

In 2015, *Cell Metabolism* published a study in which a smartphone app was used to record people's eating patterns; researchers made some interesting discoveries. They noticed that people ate for more than fifteen hours during a day and only fasted while they were in bed (which in this case was around eight or nine hours). When researchers intervened by reducing the feeding window from fourteen hours to ten or eleven hours, the results were remarkable. The participants lost weight, slept better, and had improved energy. Considering weight gain, poor sleep, and fatigue are struggles faced by many who work 24/7, these results are pretty profound [23].

Now I want to reiterate that the participants did not restrict their calories, nor did they limit the food they ate. All they did was slightly reduce the length of time that they were eating.

So while we may not be able to beat our biology, which includes the internal body clock, we can certainly work with it to help mitigate some of the effects of working 24/7. This includes being mindful of when and how often we eat.

2. Curb Sugar Cravings with Healthy Fats and Protein

One of the consequences of sleep deprivation is that it causes us to get the munchies and crave all of the bad stuff at all different times of the day. As a shift worker, I'm sure you can relate. The sweets, lollies, doughnuts, greasy hamburgers, fries: all those wonderful not-so-healthy things end up causing havoc on our waistline, particularly if we're eating them day after day, month after month, year after year.

When we crave something, it's also incredibly hard to hold back. That apple we packed in our lunchbox is by no means as appealing as the cheesecake someone generously brought into work to share. The same applies to the home-made salad. All our best efforts to eat more greens can come crashing down in an instant if we walk past the staff cafeteria and the smell of those greasy potato chips lures us in, under some kind of magnetic spell!

Sigh. There goes another diet, for the umpteenth time.

To curb these cravings (and hunger), one of the things we need to do is re-educate our taste buds. We need to replace the high-calorie, highly refined, and highly processed foods (which often are laden with addictive sugar and sugar-like substances) with more wholesome, balanced snacks. Whole foods, a selection of healthy fats, protein, and unrefined carbohydrates, will keep us feeling full, along with stabilising those blood sugar levels, which can trigger the food cravings in the first place.

Unrefined carbohydrates, which include whole grains, fruits, vegetables, and greens, are minimally processed and rich in vitamins, minerals, and fibre. They are also digested and absorbed more slowly, which produces a steady increase in blood glucose levels, which is easier for our body to tolerate [24]. This is even more important, as we just discussed in the previous section, when eating during the night.

In contrast, highly refined and processed carbohydrates such as white bread, chips, and soft drinks get absorbed very quickly, which produces an abnormal spike in our blood glucose levels, leading to hyperglycemia. In other words, an excess of blood glucose. This prompts the body to produce insulin to help with the uptake of glucose into the cells; however, this excess insulin can lead to a slump in glucose levels soon after, known as hypoglycemia. This bouncing up and down of our blood sugar and insulin levels leads to a rollercoaster ride of energy highs and lows, which is not ideal when we're already running on little sleep [24].

One trick to curb these cravings is to eat foods that are going to keep you feeling fuller for longer because, let's face it, sometimes we never know if or when we're going to get our next meal break.

> *Eat more foods that are going to keep you feeling fuller for longer.*

In other words, it all comes down to getting more bang for your meal-break buck.

Eating a high-protein meal at the start of your shift is a great way to do this (whether that's an early, late, or night shift), as it will help to lower levels of ghrelin (the hunger hormone which makes our tummy growl), which will leave you feeling more satisfied and less hungry. For example, Greek yoghurt is higher in protein and lower in sugar than regular yoghurt and is super creamy to taste. It's also a great source of calcium, B vitamins, and beneficial bacteria to support the gut. Eggs are also a great source of high-quality protein, with one large egg containing around 6 grams. They are very filling and score high on a scale called the satiety index, which measures the feeling of fullness and loss of appetite that occurs after eating [25].

Healthy fats are also one of the best satiety foods, but don't panic; fat will not make you fat. That whole fat-is-bad-for-us theory was completely misleading, based on inaccurate science. Unrefined fats are healthy and very high in energy, which leads to a reduction in appetite and subsequent intake of calories. This is a good thing when you're trying to manage your weight. Examples of healthy fats include nuts, seeds, and avocados, so having a guacamole dip on hand is an excellent way to curb those mid-shift munchies, as opposed to reaching for a sugar-laden chocolate bar from the vending machine [26] [27].

Other examples to help curb those cravings include home-made hummus dip or guacamole with capsicum, carrot or celery sticks, organic Medjool dates stuffed with nut butter, or half an avocado on toasted gluten-free bread, sprinkled with hemp seeds. These snacks will help fill the void, per se, along with providing you with an energy boost without the energy slump soon after.

3. Quench Your Thirst With Water, Not Sugar

Human beings evolved to drink water, as opposed to soft drinks, energy drinks, and even fruit juice. It's because water makes up to 60 percent of our body weight, making it critical for life. Every cell, tissue, and organ requires water to function, as it helps to carry nutrients and other material (such as blood cells and lymph) throughout the body and is essential in the elimination of waste products.

But when we replace this beautiful liquid with sugar-sweetened beverages such as soft drinks and energy drinks, it's like adding a spoon full of sugar (or more) each time we take a gulp. Yikes. I can almost feel my pants becoming tighter just thinking about this. Energy drinks, in particular, are a popular beverage for shift workers, given their high caffeine content. However, the added sugar can contribute to that expanding waistline quite quickly, particularly if we're drinking lots of them over an extended period.

We also need to keep in mind that a lot of the so-called healthy drinks, such as store-bought fruit juices and smoothies, can be loaded with heaps of sugar, which is why the absolute best way to quench our thirst is through drinking more water.

The so-called diet drinks that have been marketed to us as low-sugar options are not doing us any favours, either. This was illustrated in a study where subjects who drank diet soda (no, that was not a typo: diet soda) gained almost triple the amount of abdominal fat over nine years versus those who didn't drink soda [28].

Crazy stuff, isn't it?

On the other hand, studies have consistently shown that reducing consumption of sugary drinks leads to weight loss [29]. So keep drinking that water if you're serious about weight loss because the proof is in the pudding (or, in this case, the water). Not to mention, the fatigue-boosting benefits of upping your water intake can be a game changer for anyone working 24/7.

Don't Like the Taste of Water?

If it's water straight out of the tap, I don't blame you. Most tap water tastes pretty ordinary, and it's likely contaminated with a whole host of pollutants, including heavy metals such as lead and copper, which is why investing in a water filter is an absolute must.

To help enhance the taste, but without all the weight-inducing properties of soda and energy drinks, try adding some chopped fruit and herbs, such as watermelon, mint, citrus fruits, pineapple, cucumber, basil; the possibilities are endless. Not only will it give your water a refreshing twist, but it will help steer you in the right direction towards your ultimate goal of weight loss.

Healthy Shift Worker Action Steps

1. Eat minimally when your digestive system is sleeping.
2: Curb the cravings with healthy fat and protein.
3: Quench your thirst with water, not sugar.

Struggle 3: Feelings of Stress, Anxiety, and Depression

---

*"Stress doesn't mean that you are a failure.
It means that you are a human".*
—Dr Rangan Chatterjee

"I can't keep doing this anymore." Those were the words I said to my husband back in June 2006, after returning home one day from an early shift.

I walked through the front door, removed my shoes, sat down on the floor of our study, and proceeded to curl up into a ball and cry. I was physically, mentally, and emotionally exhausted and could barely string two words together.

My husband came into the room, wrapped his supportive arms around me, and asked, "What's wrong?"

"I just can't keep doing this anymore," I replied.

After eight months of constant stress as a result of ongoing staff shortages, coupled with a chronically sleep deprived body, I was spent.

My body was shutting down, and I had nothing left to give.

But it wasn't only me.

The ongoing stress eventually led more than a hundred people to resign over eighteen short months. An enormous number, given our workforce encompassed around three hundred people at the time.

But that day in 2006 was my tipping point.

As I stood behind one of the check-in counters at the airport that morning, looking back towards my supervisor, who was just a few meters away, I witnessed something I'd never seen before.

It was 0430, and we had a huge queue of close to one hundred people in front of us. With twenty-one counters and just four staff on shift, people were standing in lines with no one to assist them. Understandably, they were getting angry and agitated, as flights were closing for check-in, leaving them stranded.

This scene, however, was not a one-off.

Similar scenes had been playing out for eight months prior. Day after day, month after month, with little staff and huge workloads, not to mention having to do so on little sleep, amplified those feelings of stress even further.

Minimal staff and huge workloads on little sleep, amplifying those feelings of stress even further.

As I looked down towards my supervisor, I witnessed something I'll never forget. He began to act in a way that was completely out of character. He was sharp towards people, and he looked as though he was close to his breaking point.

The unrelenting stress, compounded with ongoing sleep deprivation, had slowly worn him down to the very core.

The job (and the circumstances behind it) were quite literally changing him.

It was changing all of us.

We were dropping like flies from exhaustion.

That's why, from that moment onwards, I knew I had to do something.

It's as if someone had flicked a switch inside me triggering my survival instinct, for the sake of my physical, mental, and emotional well-being.

> *It was if someone had flicked a switched inside of me triggering my survival instinct.*

After coming home and collapsing on the floor that day, I knew I'd reached a point. I had to do something I'd never done before: I had to take time off work.

It was the lowest point in my career; I had worked shift work for well over ten years without a hitch, and here I was, having to take time off work for stress.

How could that even be? I mean, what was wrong with me? Why was I no longer coping? I actually felt a tinge of guilt at the time for even taking time off work for stress; it just seemed incomprehensible that it had reached this point.

But the ongoing stress, coupled with lack of sleep, was just not sustainable.

We were being stretched and stretched like an elastic band, on the brink of snapping.

> *The ongoing stress, coupled with lack of sleep, was just not sustainable.*

I loved my job, though, and was determined not to let external circumstances dictate my future. So from that day forward, I decided to put my health first. Not only my physical health but my mental and emotional health too, because you cannot pour from an empty cup; you have to take care of yourself first.

So I did.

Does This Sound Familiar?

Given numerous workplaces these days are running on minimal staff, I'm going to assume that many of you reading this book will be able to relate to my story in some way, shape or form. I also want to highlight how working shift work can not only be stressful in itself, but it can be compounded further when the workplace becomes stressful too. I'm sure you can appreciate that it's hard enough to peel yourself out of bed at the very uncivilised hour of 3 a.m. or work through the night, but when our jobs become stressful too, it becomes a whole different ball game.

Straight away, I'm thinking paramedics, nurses, doctors, veterinarians, vet nurses, police officers, firefighters; you know who you are.

Quite simply, working shift work is stressful on our body due to frequent disruptions to our circadian rhythms or our natural sleep/wake cycle, and that's even before we've stepped foot into a stressful workplace.

> *Working shift work is stressful on our body due to continual disruption to our sleep/wake cycle, and that's even before we've stepped foot into a stressful workplace.*

And I do mean stress. Biological stress, on a cellular level, because our bodies are not designed to function in this way.

We're diurnal creatures, not nocturnal. That is, we're designed to be up during the day and asleep during the night.

But as shift workers, we don't function this way.

We work night shifts, early shifts, late shifts, split shifts, or even double shifts, which causes our body to be under constant stress. We also live in a stressful world, with so many commitments and responsibilities that our lives have become increasingly complex and demanding. So when we add shift work into an already stressful life, it can be a hazardous combination.

Working irregular hours also puts our body clocks out of sync, making us even more vulnerable to stress and burnout, as opposed to our day shift or 9–5 working cousins who can go to bed and get up at the same time every day.

What Exactly Is Stress?

Stress is a natural part of life; it's unavoidable. It can also be useful at the right dose and frequency. However, at the wrong dose and frequency, in the case of ongoing chronic stress (as opposed to the more short-term acute stress), it can be damaging to our health. This is because it increases the allostatic load (or wear-and-tear) on our body, which steadily erodes our coping mechanisms over time.

It also shifts our mitochondrial function (remember the tiny organelles in our cells responsible for producing energy, or more specifically, adenosine triphosphate, otherwise known as ATP) out of energy-producing mode and into something called cell defence mode. This is not good, especially for shift workers, because when our mitochondria are operating in this mode, they're unable to produce energy, adding to our fatigue levels even more [1].

In other words, it's not only sleep deprivation that depletes our energy levels; so too does stress, and in a big way.

That being said, we know that stress is a complex phenomenon, and we all have different degrees of tolerance to it, depending on our background and personality [2], but if we work shift work, and our job is stressful too, then things need to change and change quickly.

By definition, stress is a "stimulus which evokes a stress response" which endangers or perceives to threaten our survival. The key word here being *perceive*. It is our perception of a stressful event (whether it's real or we perceive it to be real) which triggers the same response in our body [2]. For example, being chased by a wild elephant is going to initiate a stress response, but so too can an alarm clock piercing the silence of our bedroom at 3 a.m. or signing into our computer and seeing fifty unanswered emails.

All three of these situations can cause us to flinch or panic, depending on how we see or perceive them.

Now, an alarm clock and countless emails are way less stressful than being chased by a wild elephant.

I agree, but incredibly, our body doesn't know the difference.

It responds in the same way, whether it's an elephant, an alarm clock, or a bucket load of emails.

And here's the kicker:

Our body is designed to deal with an occasional bit of stress, but in today's world, we no longer have these one-off encounters with wild elephants. We're facing a herd of wild elephants (alarm clocks and emails), day after day, causing us to continually be on high alert as we endeavour to keep ourselves safe. Essentially, we're unable to turn the dial towards the off position, which is causing us to burn out way faster than our ancestors did before us.

Our body responds by either fighting or fleeing from the wild elephant, alarm clock, or emails, which involves activating the hypothalamic-pituitary-adrenal (HPA) axis, causing a cascade of biochemical reactions to occur in the body. At the same time, all this is happening: the digestive, reproductive, and immune systems are all shut down because digesting a hamburger, making a baby, or fighting a virus isn't exactly a high priority when being chased by a wild elephant [3].

Now I want to focus on the letter A of the HPA axis, which stands for adrenal glands, because they bear the brunt of our stress. Ironically, compared to other organs, they're tiny, the size of a walnut, but in today's high-pressured, high-paced world, the adrenal glands are getting thrashed. It's as though there's a tiny person straddled atop each kidney, holding a whip in hand, ready to charge out the gates to start a race that has no finish line.

Once the adrenal glands receive a message from the pituitary gland in the form of adrenocorticotrophic hormone (yes, another one of those long-winded, hard-to-pronounce words; call it ACTH), it stimulates the adrenals to produce adrenalin and cortisol. Each time cortisol is produced, it initiates the release of blood sugar, which is needed in the muscles to help us run away from the wild elephant, the alarm clock, and fifty unanswered emails. This then prompts the pancreas to release insulin, which is needed to help move blood sugar into cells of the muscles as a source of energy, enabling us to safely run from these impending threats.

But here lies the problem.

We don't actually need to run away from our alarm clocks. Okay, we might be tempted to throw it out the window, but we just have to hit a button (maybe a couple of times, if you love the snooze button like me).

The same thing applies if we're sitting at our desk, replying to heaps of unanswered emails, or working on the triage desk in the emergency department of a hospital. As we begin to feel stressed, glucose starts to build up in the body, but it's not getting used up. In other words, it has nowhere to go.

So where does it end up?

In our fat cells or adipose tissue, which, interestingly, congregates mainly around our belly, as the body's way of helping to protect our organs from stress. They quite literally cushion them with extra fat.

So not only does ongoing stress cause the adrenal glands to become burnt out from having to continually produce adrenalin and cortisol, but this excess cortisol can lead to insulin resistance (a common trait in shift workers) and the promotion

> *Excess cortisol can lead to insulin resistance and the promotion of fat deposits around the abdominal area.*

of fat deposits around the abdominal area. This beer belly or apple-shaped pattern of weight gain increases our risk of heart disease and type 2 diabetes, along with a host of other chronic conditions, highlighting some of the dangers of long-term stress [4]. The correlation of high levels of the stress hormone cortisol and increased body mass index (BMI) was confirmed in a 2011 study comparing the cortisol levels in the scalp hair of shift workers, versus those who worked day shifts [5].

Why Are Shift Workers So Vulnerable?

*"We can't always control what happens to us,
but we can always control how we respond to what happens to us".*
—Victor Frankl

First and foremost, we need to recognise that lack of sleep is a form of physiological stress; shift workers have to endure this week after week, month after month, year after year, which is not ideal. According to circadian neuroscientist Russell Foster, tired people are massively stressed due to constant sleep deprivation, which can lead to memory loss, suppressed immunity, high blood pressure, and higher rates of cancer [6].

Animal studies have also shown that long-term stress and nocturnal sleep deprivation, typically associated with shift work, impacts on our gastrointestinal health in many ways, including altering the delicate balance of the gut microbiome or microbiota, which can lead to an overgrowth of pathogenic bacteria, which can lead to intestinal permeability, or leaky gut syndrome [7].

Stress also decreases gut motility or bowel movement by diverting blood flow away from the gastrointestinal tract towards our muscles, enabling us to run away from those emails, which, in survival terms, is way more important than digesting the last meal we ate.

What's particularly concerning, however, is how stress and lack of sleep can make us susceptible to mental health disorders, such as anxiety and depression. A study published in the journal *SLEEP* identified a link between low serotonin and shift workers who worked rotational shifts [8]. Serotonin is a hormone and neurotransmitter that is often referred to as our happy hormone; it plays an essential role in the regulation of sleep, along with being associated with anger, depression, and anxiety if levels are low.

Boost Your Resilience to Shift Work Stress

So when we work shift work, our body is in a state of biological stress, whether we feel stressed or not. Many people also operate under some pretty stressful work conditions, whether that's due to time or financial constraints, or from having to save someone from a burning car.

It's for this very reason we need to place a considerable focus and emphasis on calming and restoring the nervous system to help reduce your likelihood of developing long-term, stress-related health conditions later on. In other words, you not only need to embrace the concept of self-care when working 24/7, you need to take it to a whole new level.

While we cannot always control the stress in our workplace, nor the havoc sleep deprivation places on our health, we can undoubtedly implement ways to help manage our stress so that the health implications are less severe. This topic is so important, which is why, after much deliberation, I decided to include six tips, all of which are designed to help improve your shift work resilience and minimise those feelings of stress, anxiety, and depression.

1. Start Going into Work in an Imaginary Bubble

I know what you're thinking. *Going into work in an imaginary what Audra? Have you completely lost your mind?!*

I totally get that your initial instinct would be to support the theory of yes, I have indeed lost my mind. But please hear me out.

Because this simple act of going into work in an 'imaginary bubble' was a real game-changer for me. It quite literally helped me to cope with all of the external stresses that were playing out in my workplace at the time.

> *While I knew I couldn't change what was happening in my workplace, I knew I had the power to change how I responded to it.*

While I knew I couldn't change what was happening in my workplace, what I did know, is that I had the power to change how I responded to it.

It meant coming up with a different strategy. One which included imagining I had some kind of protective shield surrounding me; keeping me safe from harm each time I set foot in what was, at the time, an incredibly stressful and toxic work environment.

Remarkably, this simple act had the most calming effect on my nervous system. I felt less anxious and was able to stay focused on what I was there to do. That being to provide the best customer service possible to all those who walked through those airport terminal doors.

Funnily enough, when I mentioned this to a work colleague, he replied with a "Can I jump in your bubble with you?!"

My response was "Um, no. Get your own bubble!" providing both of us with a bit of a giggle.

So whilst this recommendation may come across as a little bit left-field, please be open to trying it. I can honestly say it made a huge difference in how I was able to deal with all of the ongoing workplace stress that, let's face it, should never have occurred in the first place.

I will be forever grateful that I came across this idea (to this day, I have no idea where or how) but hope by sharing it, it may help others who are going through similar stressful situations in their own workplace.

2. Embrace the Concept of Saying No

Another strategy that I began to implement when I felt as though everything was getting on top of me, and when I was feeling so overworked and unhappy, was learning to say no. And doing so without feeling any obligation to explain my reasons why.

To take charge of our health, we need to put ourselves first, which for a lot of mums and dads out there is a hard concept to embrace.

Shift workers don't just burn the candle at both ends; we set the bit in the middle on fire as well.

But we cannot take care of those around us if we're neglecting to take care of ourselves first. It's near impossible.

I'm sure you're familiar with the phrase "burning the candle at both ends." Well, shift workers don't just burn the candle at both ends; we set the bit in the middle on fire as well.

This is because we keep pushing our bodies to do way more than what they're designed to do, forcing them to work against their natural circadian rhythm or sleep/wake cycle, day after day, week after week, year after year.

Because we can.

Well, let me rephrase that: Our bodies allow us to do so, for a while, anyway.

But when we commit to so many things and people (many of whom are not working shift work), it's only a matter of time before that burning candle turns into a melted mess, and there's no way back. We essentially become physically and emotionally depleted to our very core.

It can happen during various times throughout our career, but when we've reached a point of burn-out, when our cortisol levels have flatlined because our adrenal glands have quite literally run out of puff, this is not good.

So before things become this dire, let's start putting on the brakes. Let's slow things down by reducing your sensory load, so you feel less stressed, and you don't become a train wreck.

The best place to start is by learning to say no more often (and yes, this does include saying no to overtime); but more importantly, you must be okay with saying no. In other words, learn to say no without justification, because the reality is, you don't have to justify your decisions to anyone.

When you begin to get into the habit of putting yourself first and learning to say, "Thank you, but no," more often, your workload will drop, and your levels of stress and anxiety will begin to dissipate.

I remember coming across a beautiful quote by Courtney Carver, the founder of Be More with Less, an organisation dedicated to helping people simplify their life so that they can really live, and it went like this:

> "I don't say no because I am so busy. I say no because I don't want to be so busy."
> —Courtney Carver

"I don't say no because I am so busy. I say no because I don't want to be so busy."

Because being busy is overrated. I've never understood why the term *busyness* has morphed into some kind of badge of honour, as though it's a good thing.

But I don't get it.

What's so great about being busy all of the time? It only leads to burnout, even more so if you're combining it with working shifts and running on little sleep.

It also accelerates our aging and, more importantly, takes all the fun out of living a fulfilling life, so I don't see the benefits here.

Alternatively, by reducing your schedule, you will begin to notice your stress and anxiety levels drop substantially, which is precisely what a biologically stressed-out shift worker needs.

3. Go Easy on the Cups of Stress (Coffee and Energy Drinks)

I know, I know, just like I mentioned in struggle number 1 about prioritising your sleep, you probably want to throw this book at me for even suggesting that you go easy on the coffee and energy drinks. But trust me, your adrenal glands do not like coffee (or more specifically, caffeine). This is because every time you consume a caffeinated beverage, it's like drinking a cup of stress.

'It's like drinking a cup of what, Audra?"

Just stick with me here, and I promise it will all make sense shortly.

You see, the thing is, caffeine

> *Every time you consume a caffeinated drink, it's like you are drinking a cup of stress.*

triggers the adrenal glands to produce the stress hormones adrenalin and cortisol, which, in turn, causes a spike in your blood sugar to provide you with the energy to flee from an impending threat.

Remember the wild elephant? Essentially, each time you drink a cup of caffeine, whether it's in the form of coffee, tea, soda, or energy drinks, it triggers the same cascading response of hormones as if faced with that wild elephant. In other words, it fires you up in the same way.

It also explains why you often crave sugar when you're under stress. It's the body's way of telling you that you need energy (in the form of glucose) to give you strength to run away from the impending threat (real or imagined).

But here's what's important to know: Caffeine does not actually cure your tiredness per se; it just tricks the body into thinking that it's not tired.

It covers up your tiredness by latching onto the adenosine receptors in the brain that are responsible for making you feel tired in the first place. Now, this is not a problem if you're an occasional coffee or caffeinated beverage drinker, but if you drink it daily, especially in the form of multiple cups of coffee or energy drinks, these adenosine receptors begin to change and adapt. Over time, this leads to a caffeine tolerance, where you require more caffeine to get the same stimulatory effect, as well as an energy crash when the caffeine begins to wears off [9]. Not an ideal scenario for anyone running on low batteries of energy at the best of times.

So I have an alternative. It's going to improve your energy, decrease your feelings of stress, and help reduce your expanding waistline too.

A study undertaken on chronically sleep-deprived women who were getting less than six and a half hours of sleep per night, showed how ten minutes of walking up and down stairs proved to be much more energising than ingesting 50 milligrams of caffeine [10]. Given most workplaces are multistory and come with plenty of stairs, allocating ten minutes of walking up and down stairs will not only provide you with a much-needed energy boost and alleviate some of your feelings of stress, it will also help to burn off some of that surging glucose that is swirling around in your blood. In excess, it turns into that fat-around-the-belly so many of us are desperately trying to avoid.

Now I'm by no means suggesting that you need to eradicate caffeine (although that would be beneficial). I get it that most of us like to have the odd cup to get us through our shift; I know I certainly did. All I'm suggesting is that you consider reducing the amount that you drink; ideally, have one cup at the start of your shift and replace the remaining with more movement and water.

You could also alternate the coffee with green tea or matcha, which contains a compound called L-theanine, which helps to reduce some of the jitteriness and decreased blood flow to the brain which often occurs after consuming coffee [11]. Even adding fat into our coffee, such as butter or MCT oil (short for medium-chain triglyceride oil), and drinking herbal tonics have become increasingly popular, as the fat can provide the brain with a source of energy, while certain types of herbs, such as medicinal mushrooms, can support the adrenal glands during times of stress [12] [13]. In other words, they're helping to buffer the effects of caffeine when it's consumed on its own.

It's all about implementing a common-sense approach when it comes to consuming caffeine, because while it's going to perk you up temporarily, the adverse effects on your nervous system, mood, and cognitive function, especially when you're consuming lots of it, are going to be much more long-lasting.

4. Do More of What Makes You Happy

As adults, I think we're all guilty at times of falling into the trap of constant work mode and forgetting to do more of what brings us joy. You may even think you're not worthy of having joy in your life, due to having so many responsibilities.

Well, I'm here to tell you that you absolutely are. Shift work can take its toll, so having a release valve, in the form of doing more things that are enjoyable to you, is going to do wonders for your mental health and well-being. It's also a great distraction if things (or people) at work are pushing your buttons a little, if you know what I mean.

> *Doing more of what makes you happy is not being selfish; it's a necessity.*

I want to point out that doing more of what makes you happy is not being selfish; it's a necessity. It's about being kind to yourself, just as you are to other people.

If you're in a state of chronic stress (unfortunately, this is the case for many who work 24/7), it's only a matter of time before it's going to manifest in illness later on, unless we do all we possibly can to help reduce some of those risks.

Investing time in yourself and having fun, is going to help release some of that pent-up stress, whether it's physical or emotional, which will enable you to be in a much better position to help others. It's a win-win all around.

So while life can get busy, I think it's essential to do one thing (or more) each week that brings you joy and makes you feel good. Maybe this means reacquainting yourself with a hobby or taking up a new one (such as playing an instrument, going dancing, attending a cooking class, learning to paint, or even immersing yourself in a flotation tank for an hour). Alternatively, it may even be as simple as going for a swim or taking yourself to the movies.

Whatever it is for you, remember to do more of what makes you happy, and spoil yourself often because you're a shift worker. You're tired; you're exhausted. You deserve to have plenty of fun and enjoyment in your life, because you are doing what most people could not or would not do. Which is why if anyone deserves to be pampered, it's a shift worker, period.

5. Increase Your Intake of Stress-Busting Nutrients and Foods

"How you think and feel is directly affected by what you eat."
—Nutritionist Patrick Holford

Whenever we are under stress, which happens often when working 24/7, the body becomes depleted in nutrients much more quickly because there's a higher demand for them. Ironically, when we do feel stressed, we tend to gravitate towards comfort foods, which usually contain lots of sugar and highly processed fats that are lacking in essential nutrients [2]. I'm sure you can think of a time (or two) when you succumbed to a bowl of ice cream or takeaway pizza after a hectic day at work.

> When we feel stressed, we tend to gravitate towards comfort foods, which contain sugar and processed fats that are lacking in essential nutrients.

The trouble with this type of eating is that it places even more stress on the body, as opposed to helping improve its resistance to stress. There are, however, specific nutrients which play an essential role in helping to reduce our stress hormones, some of which include water-soluble vitamins B and C, along with magnesium [2]. So let's have a quick chat about these critical nutrients.

Vitamin C is essential in counteracting some of the effects of stress; it does so by lowering blood pressure and cortisol. It's also critical for adrenal function (remember those little powerhouses sitting on top of our kidneys, pumping out hormones in times of stress?). For anyone working 24/7, nurturing and restoring the adrenal glands (along with our mitochondria) should be a significant focus of our health, right after improving our sleep. Foods containing vitamin C include papaya, capsicum, broccoli, spinach, brussels sprouts, blueberries, strawberries, pineapple, and the camu camu berry [14][15].

B vitamins have an essential role in the development and maintenance of our nervous system, along with helping to maintain normal blood-sugar levels that help to stabilise our mood and energy. Vitamin B5, in particular, otherwise known as pantothenic acid, is often referred to as an anti-stress vitamin, as it helps to support the adrenal glands and improve our coping mechanisms. They're also essential in helping to boost the size and number of our mitochondria, which are responsible for providing energy to our cells, along with building our resilience to stress. In other words, the fewer mitochondria we have, the lower we're able to tolerate, handle, and adapt to stress so we need to do all we can to preserve them [16]. Some of the foods that contain B-vitamins include meat, fish, broccoli, legumes, nutritional yeast, nuts, and seeds.

Magnesium is often regarded as an anti-stress mineral because it helps to relax tense muscles, balance blood sugar levels, and calm the nervous system by reducing cortisol [17]. It also helps us to sleep, which as we know can be quite elusive when working 24/7. Unfortunately, just like vitamins B and C, magnesium becomes depleted during times of stress, so maintaining our magnesium reserves is critical to buffer the effects of stress. Foods containing magnesium include avocados, nuts, seeds, legumes, leafy greens, and bananas.

Although my nutritional philosophy is always to focus on food first, given shift workers push their bodies to do something that we haven't evolved to do, I often recommend supporting the body with supplements, even just temporarily. Doing this can be instrumental in giving our sleep-deprived bodies a much-needed boost, but on a cellular level, which is what shift workers need to sustain energy, improve mitochondrial function, and increase resilience to stress.

6. Move More Regularly, but Gently

Exercise in almost every form is an excellent reliever of stress, as it helps the body to produce endorphins, which are our feel-good, happy hormones [18]. When we get this influx of endorphins zooming around our body, it helps to boost our mood, along with reducing feelings of stress and anxiety [19]. Sounds like the perfect kind of therapy for a biologically stressed-out shift worker, don't you think?

While I'm not suggesting that we do this right in the middle of our shift (although that would be awesome), most people need to be incorporate more movement into their daily lives.

Some of you may find pounding the treadmill or doing a high-intensity workout at the gym beneficial in alleviating your stress, particularly after a crazy day at work, but I have to say, I'm more in favour of something a little more gentle. Things like yoga, qigong, and meditation can help calm your nervous system down, as opposed to firing it up even more.

Now before you say "But Audra, I'm so not a yoga person, and I can't meditate," stick with me here because just saying that tells to me that you probably need it more than you think. What I mean by this is, if you are a Type A personality and are very driven and hyperactive, then your body (in particular, your adrenal glands and mitochondria) may be desperately craving for you to slow down. If this resonated with you, you're probably like an Energizer Bunny who keeps going and going. That is, of course, until your body eventually forces you to stop, from chronic fatigue and exhaustion.

Restorative yoga and meditation are great at helping to support a tired and wired body; this form of practice usually incorporates diaphragmatic breathing, which we touched on in chapter 1, which helps to calm a frazzled nervous system. It does so by moving our body out of sympathetic, fight-or-flight dominance (being chased by wild elephants, alarm clocks, and emails) and into the much more calming and nurturing "rest and digest" or parasympathetic arm of our nervous system. If you are a "go, go, go" kind of person, this won't be easy (a conversation that I've had with many of my Super Mum, I-Can-Do-Everything clients), but it's even more critical that you slow down.

Some of you reading this book right now might be thinking, *But I need the high-intensity stuff. I need to pound on the treadmill for hours to get rid of all my stress.*

For sure, I get it.

I'm not discounting the benefits of other forms of exercise such as high-intensity interval training. Quite the contrary, as we need to be including a variety of activities, especially those that get our heart rates pumping. But I think it's important to acknowledge that while we may feel amazing after a high-intensity workout, each time you do this, you're adding even more stress (and cortisol) to an already stressed-out and depleted body. Especially if you're someone who goes straight to the gym after night-shift.

In contrast, moderate to low-intensity exercises such as yoga, qigong, and tai chi do not cause a significant increase in cortisol levels [20]. Instead, they help to calm us down, as opposed to winding us up, which can be so incredibly beneficial for anyone working 24/7.

Bonus Tip: Ask for Help

"Asking for help is always a sign of strength."
—Michelle Obama

Shift work can be a pretty challenging occupation, in more ways than one. We're also under a lot more pressure these days, whether it's due to time or financial constraints, or if the actual job comes with a considerable amount of responsibility, such as those working in the emergency services or healthcare sectors.

But when your job is stressful, *and* you're running on little sleep, it can only be a matter of time before it wears you down to the core.

I'm sure you can relate to having days when you just wanted to collapse in a heap from total exhaustion, only you couldn't. You kept soldiering on because you had to or you felt compelled to or felt a sense of responsibility, not only to your co-workers but to your family.

But I want to point out something significant:

Despite what you may think, you're not superhuman.

No one is, and there's not a single person on this planet who is. Okay, maybe Roger Federer, but I know for a fact that he really values his sleep!

It's why I feel strongly that shift workers are an elite group of individuals who are doing what most people could not, and would not, do.

So when you experience those feelings of stress, anxiety, or even depression, it's okay to acknowledge it. In fact, if you've never experienced these feelings, then maybe you are, in some unique kind of way, superhuman.

But for the majority of us, we're not immune to these conditions.

Good health doesn't just apply to our physical health. It also refers to our mental health.

So if you've reached a point where it feels as though it's all too much, please ask for help. There's nothing courageous about burning the candle at both ends (and lighting the bit in the middle), for decades on end, particularly if you've also got some serious stuff going on in your personal life. Perhaps seek out a counsellor or a psychologist who can help. I found cognitive behavioural therapy particularly beneficial when I had lots of things going on in my life. It helped me to see things differently, which in turn enabled me to respond to stressful events in a completely different (and better) way.

Healthy Shift Worker Action Steps

1. Start going into work in an imaginary bubble.
2. Embrace the concept of saying no.
3. Go easy on the cups of stress (coffee and energy drinks).
4. Do more of what makes you happy.
5. Increase your intake of stress-busting nutrients and foods.
6. Move more regularly, but gently.

Bonus tip: Ask for help.

Struggle 4: A Depleted and Burnt-Out Immune System

"Sleep is the golden chain that ties health and our bodies together."
—Thomas Dekker

One of the biggest struggles many of us encounter when working 24/7 is being prone to getting sick. I guess you could call it one of the many perks to working outside regular business hours.

When I look back on the first few years of my shift-working career, I lost count of how many times I got sick. Nothing serious, just continually getting colds, sore throats, and losing my voice, along with feeling achy and, at times, nauseous.

Of course, there were plenty of times when my sleep tank was running close to empty, but at the time, I never really put two and two together. Fast forward to 2019; I certainly have a much better appreciation of how poor sleep leads to illness and why, when we're feeling unwell, all our body wants to do is sleep. It instinctively yearns for more rest; it knows that sleep will help to heal and replenish the immune system [1].

The real kicker for shift workers is that when we work irregular hours, gaining sufficient quality sleep is not as easy as it sounds, thanks to struggle number 1: ongoing and relentless sleep deprivation and disruption.

Why Shift Workers' Immune Systems Are Compromised

Perhaps due to a combination of poorly designed rosters, unrealistic workloads, and high stress (or simply because we're trying to juggle so many things at once as our lives become increasingly busy), we tend to push ourselves to a point where our bodies never really get enough downtime to recuperate properly.

We've all heard of the saying "burning the candle at both ends," but as I've mentioned previously, I believe shift workers take this to a whole new level. We don't just burn the candle at both ends; we set fire to the bit in the middle as well.

We push and push ourselves to keep going and often ignore our body's instinct's to sleep. And we do this, for the most part, because we have to be at work.

This makes shift workers vulnerable to falling ill, as our bodies are continually in a state of fight-or-flight, survival mode, which over time takes a tremendous toll on our immune system.

Quite simply, sleep deprivation weakens our immune system, preventing it from functioning as it should, so the chances of falling ill for shift workers are much higher than for those who have a regular sleep routine [2].

The chances of falling ill are much higher for shift workers than for those who have a regular sleep routine.

In his TED talk titled "Why Do

We Sleep?" neuroscientist and circadian rhythm specialist Professor Russell Foster explains why tired people tend to have higher rates of overall infection [2].

There are various mechanisms behind this, but studies have shown that sleep deprivation reduces immunity cells, called T-cells, and increases inflammatory cells in our body called cytokines. This fundamentally alters the body's immune response and increases proinflammatory markers such as tumour necrosis factor-alpha (TNF-a), interleukin 10 (IL-10), and C-reactive protein (CRP) [3456].

What makes shift workers even more vulnerable, unlike our 9–5 non-shift-working-cousins who may at times run on little sleep, is that thanks to a mixture of early shifts and night shifts, disrupting our circadian rhythm also impairs the immune system.

So sleep deprivation, coupled with disturbed circadian rhythms, is like a double whammy for shift workers.

This is because every organ, tissue, and cell in our body is under the masterful instruction of the central body clock, otherwise known as the suprachiasmatic nucleus in the brain (yes there's that hard to pronounce word again)! Deviating from this cycle can have adverse effects on specific physiological functions in the body, including those found in the immune system [7]. Even disturbed melatonin secretion, as a result of circadian rhythm disruption (that all-important sleep-regulating hormone that also moonlights as a powerful antioxidant), can lead to a dysregulation of the immune system. The time of night or day when we sleep is also an important factor; immune cells respond to challenges much more effectively at night compared to in the morning [89]. Not the best of news if you're a permanent night shifter, but vital that you're aware of, nonetheless.

How to Boost Your Immune System while Working 24/7

A sleep-deprived body is always going to find it harder to keep its immune system healthy and robust. It's the harsh reality of the situation, and I'm not going to tell you otherwise. However, by having this awareness, you can make better dietary and lifestyle choices to help build your body's natural resistance to disease and infection, thereby minimising your chances of falling ill in the first place.

It's important to note, that when you do get sick, it's an indication that your body is run down and no longer coping. So make sure you listen to all the signals your body is giving you, rather than ignoring them. Honour it with sufficient rest so it can heal and recover much more quickly.

1. Prioritise Your Sleep: Take Two

"Sleep is a fundamental human need that must be respected".
—Arianna Huffington

Sounding familiar? Yup. Here we go again. I've got my "you must prioritise your sleep" hat on again because, as you've just read, sleep is one of the most important tools our body has to help support the immune system. Quite simply, its level of significance cannot be underestimated.

As I touched on in chapter 1, while the concept of prioritising our sleep might sound obvious, so many of us fail to do so, even when working 24/7.

We're up late at night, spending countless hours on our electronic devices, along with staring aimlessly into the glowing screens of tablets or flat-screen TVs. Maybe you regularly go out partying into the wee hours of the morning, despite having an early shift the next day, or you're mindlessly scrolling the internet when you know you should be sleeping. If this is the case, please don't fool yourself into thinking you don't need much sleep.

> *Please don't fool yourself into thinking you don't need much sleep.*

Clinical trials have illustrated that without sufficient sleep, infection-fighting antibodies and cells become depleted and are no longer able to protect you from infection [10]. In other words, your entire immune system is dependent on sleep to keep you well.

So if we combine a disrupted sleeping pattern with poor lifestyle habits, choices, and behaviours, such as taking our sleep for granted, it's like adding fuel to an already smouldering fire.

> *Taking our sleep for granted is like adding fuel to an already smouldering fire.*

So please, please, prioritise your sleep, especially when working 24/7, because your body relies heavily on the immune-enhancing qualities of sleep to keep you well. Facebook, Instagram, and Netflix will all be there in the morning, I promise!

2. Nourish Your Gut by Eating More Veggies

*"Well-functioning gut flora is the major regulator
and housekeeper of our immune system."*
—Dr Natasha Campbell-McBride.

I'm going to put forward a question to you, and I want you to be brutally honest in your answer. How many vegetables do you include in your diet every single day?

The reason I ask is that vegetables are essentially Mother Nature's little packages of nutritional goodness, designed exclusively to help fuel your immune system so your body can thrive.

Despite the incredible immune boosting superpowers of vegetables and fruits, a staggering 96 percent of Australian adults are not consuming the recommended five servings of vegetables and two servings of fruit per day. That's a pretty woeful and somewhat embarrassing statistic, given we live in a country that has an abundant supply of fresh produce [11].

Perhaps those statistics are similar to where you live too.

Now you might be asking, how do vegetables (or more specifically, plant-based foods) help keep you healthy?

Well, before I answer that question, I want to point out something that, deep down, you probably already know. Shift workers are at risk of developing a weakened immune system purely from having a consistently poor

Shift workers are at risk of developing a weakened immune system purely from having a consistently poor diet.

diet. It's the whole Catch-22 scenario where we become so tired that we lose our mojo to cook (if it was ever there in the first place), and so we reach for whatever is the quickest or most accessible, which is not always the healthiest.

But this is not doing you or your immune system any favours because consuming foods which contain little fibre and nutrients, as found in fast foods, cakes, confectionary, and most pre-packaged foods, weakens our body's ability to fend off germs and diseases. It quite literally contributes to the destruction of your immune system [12].

In contrast, plant-based foods such as whole fruits and vegetables provide your body with the fuel to keep you healthy. This is because 80 percent of our immune system is located in the lining of our gut or gastrointestinal tract, which is home to millions of microscopic bugs, otherwise known as our gut microbiome. They are instrumental in helping to keep you well. The gut microbiome help to manufacture essential nutrients such as vitamins B and K, along with producing short-chain fatty acids such as butyrate, which help to reduce inflammation and maintain the integrity of the lining of the gut. Keeping the gut lining intact is super important, as it forms a protective barrier from the outside world, preventing toxic substances from entering the bloodstream and triggering an immune response [13].

The challenge for shift workers, as I've mentioned previously, is that ongoing sleep deprivation or circadian rhythm disturbance has been shown to impair the gut lining and contribute to a disruption in the diversity of these gut bugs, leading to intestinal permeability, otherwise known as gut leakiness. This is when food particles that wouldn't ordinarily be able to squeeze through end up entering the bloodstream and triggering that immune response [14][15].

So to protect and preserve your immune system, taking care of your gut—or more specifically, the millions of tiny bugs that reside there—has to be one of your biggest priorities in building your immune defence.

This begins by eating more whole, plant-based foods to help the good gut bugs get on with their job of protecting you from nasty pathogens that want to make you sick.

These gut bugs can't do their job if they're starving, because just like you and I, they need food to function, and this is what happens when your diet consists predominantly of highly refined, prepackaged, and processed food. Studies have shown that diets high in unhealthy fats and low in fermentable fibre lead to a significant die-off in beneficial gut bacteria including bifidobacteria and butyrate-producing firmicutes and bacteriodetes [16].

> *Diets high in unhealthy fats and low in fermentable fibre lead to a significant die-off in beneficial bacteria.*

Also, a separate study published in the journal *PLOS One* demonstrated how a high-fat, high-sugar diet, combined with circadian rhythm disruption, led to intestinal dysbiosis. This is when the bad bugs outnumber the good ones, which can lead to inflammation, the key driver behind many chronic health conditions we see today [14].

And it gets worse.

An animal study published in the journal *Cell* showed that when microbes in the digestive tract (which is just the fancy term for gut bugs) don't get enough natural fibre from the food you eat, they begin to munch on the layer of mucus that lines the gut. Yes, you read that correctly. They quite literally start to eat you, causing tiny microscopic holes that allow for invading bacteria to infect the wall of your gut, the very thing that is designed to protect you from harm [17].

So it's all about building up your gut diversity, which in simple terms means having a cross-section of different types of microbes/gut bugs and ensuring the bad bugs don't outnumber the good ones. This starts by feeding them sufficient fibre, which is the non-digestible portion of plant foods; fibre provides food for the good bugs so they can get on with the job of keeping you healthy, literally from the inside out.

Now you might be asking, how can you get more veggies into your diet or, more specifically, feed those friendly gut bugs so that not only they can thrive, but you can too?

> *Throw a grated zucchini into your smoothie; it might sound strange, but trust me, this works a treat.*

The key is to avoid overanalysing. Don't complicate things. While your gut bugs are particularly fond of foods which are high in resistant starch (meaning they're resistant to digestion), such as lady finger bananas, garlic, onions, asparagus, potatoes, and legumes [16], we shouldn't be stopping there.

Consuming five servings of vegetables and two servings of fruit per day will change the diversity of your gut microbiome and give your fledgling immune system a much-needed boost.

Here are some creative ways to get more vegetables into your diet:

- Make a conscious effort to add an extra serving of vegetable at each meal. For example, a portion of asparagus at lunch and a few broccoli florets at dinner.
- Healthy snack options include home-made dips made from vegetables, such as roasted capsicum dip (which is also high in vitamin C), pumpkin, beets, and olives; use veggie sticks instead of crackers to scoop out the goodness.
- Add vegetables to your meal by grating carrots, zucchini, parsnip, or pumpkin into a bolognese sauce.
- Add a grated zucchini into your smoothie. It might sound strange, but trust me, this works a treat and adds some creaminess to your smoothie.
- If you're on a late shift, alternate scrambled eggs with an omelette packed with vegetables.
- Make a big batch of vegetable soup that you can freeze and take into work the next day. Soups are a great form of liquid nutrition that I recommend for night-shifters, as they're easy on the digestive tract.
- Up your intake of fermented vegetables such as sauerkraut, pickles, and kimchi, which are jam-packed with beneficial probiotics or live microorganisms that help your digestive tract remain healthy.
- While they're not vegetables, stewed apples are high in polyphenols, a phytochemical found in plant-based foods that give it its colour, along with other gut healing and health-protecting benefits [18]. Stewed apples can be a

perfect little snack to have on shift with a dollop of kefir or yoghurt, and you'll find a recipe in the recipe collection at the end of the book.

- If you don't eat many veggies at all right now, get a seasonal box delivered to your door each week (preferably organic) so that it inspires you to cook. Try an assortment of different veggies so you don't get bored, and if cooking is not your forte, go online and type in your ingredients to begin searching for some recipes to try. Your taste buds, along with your friendly gut bugs and immune system, will be so thankful that you did.

3. Boost Lymphatic Flow through Exercise, Harnessing the Benefits of Rebounding

I'm sure if you're reading this book right now, I don't need to convince you that it can take monk-like discipline to peel yourself off the couch and do some exercise, particularly after finishing a string of early or night shifts, when your energy level resembles a deflated balloon.

But the thing is, exercise helps to strengthen your immune system.

Research has shown a direct link between regular physical activity and improved immune function, mainly because when we exercise, it improves our circulation, enabling immune cells to circulate more quickly throughout our body, enabling them to kill bacteria and viruses more effectively [19]. It's also been shown to reduce systemic inflammation, an underlying driver behind multiple chronic diseases, thereby lowering the risks for developing cardiovascular disease, type 2 diabetes, and dementia [20].

At the other end of the spectrum, intense or vigorous exercise may reduce immunity because it leads to a rise in cortisol and adrenaline, two stress hormones released during high-intensity exercise which can suppress the immune system [19]. Ongoing, strenuous exercise has also been shown to damage the integrity of the lining of the gut, which as we now know is instrumental in a healthy immune system, as it can cause injury to the tight-junction proteins which hold the cells together and prevent gut leakiness [21].

> It's why I'm a big advocate of keeping active and moving more, but doing so in a gentle way.

It's why I'm a big advocate of keeping active and moving more, but doing so in a more gentle way, especially when your body is subjected to the onslaught of a shift-working lifestyle. Primarily, you don't want to add even more stress to your already tired and weary body.

Low-impact exercises are going to be much more nourishing and restorative on the immune system, with low to moderate exercise being particularly beneficial for night shifters, given your body often endures extreme fatigue.

So besides walking, which is the best form of exercise for the majority of the population, given it's what human beings have evolved to do, my other favourite activity to enhance health, especially when working 24/7, is rebounding.

Rebounding, which is just a fancy way to describe jumping up and down on a mini trampoline, helps the body to rid itself of toxins by improving blood and lymphatic flow. Often referred to as the body's sewerage system, the lymphatic system is instrumental in removing toxins and helping to maintain optimal functioning of the immune system. However, it relies on physical exercise because unlike the heart, which acts as a pump for the cardiovascular system, the lymphatic system doesn't have a pump to stimulate the flow of lymph [22].

The vertical up-and-down movement of rebounding also helps the immune system become stronger as your body endures weight-bearing G forces. In other words, you're defying gravity when you jump up and down on a rebounder. This action, according to research undertaken by NASA, helps T and B lymphocytes, which are involved in the immune response, become up to five times more active [22][23][24].

Pretty profound, so definitely worthwhile hopping down to the shops to purchase a mini trampoline and give it a go. As a side note, it's a great low-impact form of exercise that is gentle on the joints and therefore suitable for most people. They're also relatively cheap to purchase and don't take up a lot of space, which is handy if you live in a small house or apartment.

Most rebounding experts recommend spending around twenty minutes a day bouncing up and down, depending on your fitness level, but this can include three- or five-minute stints to your favourite music. There are heaps of instructional videos available online to give you some workout ideas, although I like to take on the "Dance like no one is watching" approach as I plug in my iPhone and tune into some of the greatest hits of the 1980s!

That, of course, is a secret between you and me. ☺

Healthy Shift Worker Action Steps

1. Prioritise your sleep; take two.
2. Nourish the gut by eating more veggies.
3. Boost lymphatic flow through exercise, harnessing the benefits of rebounding.

Struggle 5: A Disrupted Family and Social Life, Strained Relationships, and Tension in the Workplace

----

So I've saved this one for last, not because I think it's the least important, but because I want to leave a final parting message that I hope will remain etched in your mind forever. That message being: nothing is more important than fostering healthy, happy, and harmonious relationships at home and in the workplace.

And I mean nothing.

I think we can all appreciate that, due to the disruptive nature and associated challenges with working 24/7, it's a well-known fact that shift work places an enormous strain on our physical and mental well-being and also on all those we love and cherish.

While there are singles, couples, and families who adapt well to the shift-working lifestyle, as they manage to find ways to make it work, the majority struggle to adjust to the unsociable hours of working 24/7.

I do, however, want to point out that not all workplaces are the same. Some are great at putting their employees first; others, not so much.

A lot of emotional strain has to do with the fact that when we sign up for shift work, we inadvertently

> When we sign up for shift work, we inadvertently sign our family up for shift work too.

sign our family up for shift work too. The ongoing sleep and lifestyle disruption, however, can lead to increasing tensions and erratic behaviour, which if left unchecked can inflict damage.

This is why we need to value our relationships and do whatever it takes to protect them before it's too late.

How Sleep Deprivation Affects Our Emotional Empathy

I'm sure you can remember a time when you felt so tired and exhausted that you lost patience with a family member or overreacted to a work colleague over something quite trivial. If you were to look back and reflect on your behaviour, it was most likely completely out of character; when people are tired, they tend to overreact.

We're essentially not ourselves, which can trigger us to say and do things we wouldn't ordinarily do if we had enough sleep. Sleep deprivation affects an area in our brain called the prefrontal cortex, which is involved in the regulation of our emotions and in the ability to understand someone else's perspective. In other words, sleep deprivation can make us feel less empathetic towards others, which can lead to increased tension both at home and in the workplace [1].

> When we're tired, it can trigger us to say and do things that we wouldn't ordinarily do if we had enough sleep.

This was highlighted in two separate studies. Firstly, in the *Behavioural Sleep Medicine* journal, poor sleep was associated with greater marital aggression, and in the *Journal of Experimental Psychology*, sleep loss negatively affected the mood of participants by making them angry. Even moderate amounts of sleep loss, as opposed to large quantities, can lead to an increase in anger [2][3].

This is why it's super important to be aware of those times when your sleep tank is running low; as a result, you may be feeling a bit heated under the collar. This can occur after a few long and stressful shifts, so be aware if this, as it will help you make better choices and take appropriate actions. For example, you might elect to take a nap first, instead of taking your frustrations out on a family member.

> We're better people when we've had enough sleep. We're nicer to be around, and we make better choices and decisions.

This lack of empathy and heightened mood reinforces what I've been harping on about throughout this entire book: We need to take every opportunity to prioritise our sleep. Because we're better people when we've had enough sleep; we're better human beings, we're nicer to be around, and we make better choices and decisions.

Family and Social Challenges

For many reasons, it can be challenging to fulfil domestic and family responsibilities when we work 24/7, which can undoubtedly add to the strain even more [4]. This may be due to periods of fatigue or having to sleep when everyone else is wide awake, or you may not be physically present to help out, if your job involves working away for extended periods. This is undoubtedly the case for airline crews and fly-in, fly-out workers.

Having fun is like a reward for putting up with all the difficult and demanding shifts we work.

There are countless times when we're having to decline social invitations as a result of either being at work or having to work the next day, which can be incredibly frustrating and, at times, disheartening. Having an active family and social life is our birthright, just as it is for those who work 9-5. It's essentially our reward for working hard and making a valuable contribution to society.

Never is this more evident than for those who work in the healthcare and emergency services sectors, occupations which often require working long hours, under some pretty stressful conditions, putting their own health and safety at risk to help others. So, yes, being able to enjoy some leisure time with those we love and cherish is something most of us look forward to, particularly after a run of some pretty difficult and demanding shifts.

That being said, when we work shift work, it can be tough to keep up with friends and family because we're either at work or sleeping in preparation for work.

How to Protect Your Relationships, Maintain a Social Life, and Reduce Workplace Tension

Unless we can get our friends and family to work the same shifts as us (yeah, I know; that's never going to happen), it's going to require a fair bit of give and take, along with some creative juggling and a strong will, to make it happen. The same applies when diffusing workplace tension and conflict, but like with anything, if there's a will, there's always a way.

1. Read the Book The 5 Love Languages

If there's one book every shift worker on the planet should read (besides this one, of course), it's *The 5 Love Languages* by Gary Chapman [5]. While anyone would benefit from reading this book, as it's not explicitly written for shift workers, we know there is a strong correlation between relationship strain and marriage breakdown amongst many who work irregular hours [6]. While there are many factors, if you want to learn some simple and practical strategies to help safeguard your relationship, then I cannot recommend this book highly enough.

The 5 Love Languages helps its readers learn how to have healthy, fulfilling, and meaningful relationships by recognising their love language and, more importantly, that of their spouse or partner.

These love languages fall under several categories: words of affirmation, quality time, receiving gifts, acts of service, and physical touch. As Gary states so eloquently in his book, "We must be willing to learn our spouse's primary love language if we are to be effective communicators of love." Given communication is everything, reading this book will be the best investment you ever make in your relationship, which, after all, is worth fighting for, don't you think?

2. Set Socialisation Goals to Connect, Device Free

"Paying attention to people you love is 2% effort,
and 98% not looking at your phone."
—Courtney Carver

It's 2019. We're able to connect to people all around the world via social media, but in many ways, that has driven us to become more and more disconnected. You only need to sit in a coffee shop and look around to see that people are more interested in their mobile phones than the person they're sitting next to. We've become totally disconnected.

Loneliness and social isolation can even increase our risks of mortality, so catching up with friends and family can quite literally enhance our health and well-being [7]. Pretty cool, don't you think? Human beings instinctively crave personal contact. We're essentially hardwired to connect, which is why it makes sense that relationships become strained if we don't communicate or spend quality time together.

Of course, there are going to be times when we've had a hectic and stressful day at work, and the last thing we feel like doing is talking to someone, but we should never underestimate the positive effects of being around others.

> *It feels good being around others, chatting, laughing and sharing our experiences and vice versa.*

I'm sure you would agree that it feels good chatting, laughing, and sharing experiences and vice versa. In many ways, it can invigorate us when we're feeling so tired and exhausted.

Of course, I'm not referring to friends and family who are negative or make you feel as though they drain every inch of life out of you. You need to keep those catch-ups to a minimum. I'm also not referring to spending time with friends and family on social media. In my mind, that does not count as true social time.

While social media has its benefits (I've met some incredible people all over the world, thanks to Facebook and Instagram), I'm talking about real-life connection. Connecting with people the good old-fashioned way, just like we did back in 1995 (for those of you who are old enough to remember those face-to-face, device-free days)!

Which is why I like to set some socialisation goals to connect, device free. So many of us set new year's goals to lose weight, get a new job, earn a certain amount of money, and so on. But when was the last time you set yourself a New Year (or even mid-year or end-of-year) goal to catch up with more people or to enhance your relationships?

For most people, the answer to that question is going to be "Never," which is why, from this day forward, I'd like you to do just that: set yourself some socialisation and relationship goals to connect, device free.

Now you might be thinking, *I just don't have time for that.*

Hmm. Really? You don't have time for your spouse, family, or friends? I'm pretty sure you do; it's just that you haven't made it a priority. It's why we need to schedule in the time to make it happen because if it's not scheduled, it's just not going to happen.

> *If it's not scheduled, it's just not going to happen.*

Another day, another week, another month is going to pass, and, suddenly, we've found ourselves becoming increasingly distant, lonely, and, as mentioned earlier, even angry, as we're no longer communicating. It becomes a recipe for relationship disaster.

So it's time to dig out the rosters and start organising some spouse, family, and friend time in the next thirty days, device free.

While this initial step is probably going to be the hardest (co-ordinating days and times), it all comes back to being proactive. As soon as your roster rolls out, check when your days off are, and schedule in some relationship and social time because it's easy to blame shift work for everything, including the demise of our relationships, but we all have the same amount of time. It's just what we choose to do with it.

Case Study 4. Hanging Out with Our Phones More Than Each Other

I distinctly remember a time when I was on my way to work, at the very unfriendly hour of 4 a.m., and sitting in the staff bus that takes us from the domestic airport carpark to the airport terminal.

The bus, filled with pilots, flight crew, and ground staff, felt somewhat eerie because 95 percent of the people on the bus were looking down at their phones.

A work colleague, who shall I say was of more senior years, in a way that everyone on the bus could hear, yelled out, "No one is talking to each other anymore, even at 4 a.m."

Even though it was super early and most of us were still trying to pry our eyes open and wake ourselves up, engaging in conversation through our phones appeared to be more important than connecting with those who were sitting right next to us.

It was undoubtedly a defining moment for many of us on that bus that morning, including myself.

3. Would You Like to Work with You?

"Be kind, for everyone you meet is fighting a battle you know nothing about."
—Unknown

Of course, we all want to have a harmonious family and social life, especially when working a challenging shift. But the same applies to our work life too, which is why we all need to ask ourselves this question: "Would you like to work with you?" Because when I hear of workplaces that have bullying and narcissistic behaviour, my initial response is, "Why?"

I mean, I don't get it.

Isn't working a job with odd hours hard enough without having to endure this type of school-yard behaviour? Considering our workmates are someone's mother, sister, brother, wife, or husband, shouldn't we be treating them with kindness too?

> *Our workmates are someone's mother, sister, brother, wife, or husband, shouldn't we be treating them with kindness too?*

Shouldn't we be treating others in the same way as we'd like to be treated?

Fortunately for me, I have many cherished memories that I will take away from working at the airport: all of the fun and laughs that I shared with my workmates.

Sure, there were plenty of stressful and exhausting moments, but being able to have fun at work was always high on my priority because being at work forms such a massive part of our life, and being serious and moody all the time is no fun at all.

So to help make this shift working journey sustainable (and dare I say enjoyable), we all need to come together as one and support each other any way we can. A family is, after all, not only our blood relatives but those we share a big part of our life with, which of course includes our shift working family.

Bonus Tip: Give a Copy of This Book to Your Friends, Family, and Work Colleagues

As you near the end of this book (well done for making it this far), my parting words to you are this: If it's a constant uphill battle trying to explain to your friends and family that "Yes, I am working again this weekend," or you sense a bit of tension each time you have to decline a social invitation, then give them a copy of this book.

While we're not expecting any accolades (although I've often thought we deserve an Oscar, Grammy, or some other fancy trophy for doing what we do), a little bit of compassion and understanding when we're working or catching up on some much-needed sleep would be greatly appreciated.

As a population, shift workers are some of the most misunderstood people on the planet, because shift work is not only a job, but rather a lifestyle, and one that is often worlds apart from anyone who works Monday–Friday, 9–5. So if reading this book helps to break down some of that confusion or misunderstanding, then it's going to be the best investment that your family, friends, and co-workers ever make, along with helping to create a healthy shift-worker ripple effect with all those around you.

Healthy Shift Worker Action Steps

1. Read the book *The 5 Love Languages*.
2. Set socialisation goals to connect, device free.
3. Would you like to work with you?

Bonus tip: Give a copy of this book to your friends, family, and work colleagues.

Part 4.
Conclusion

Where to from Here? The Choice Is Up to You

----

*"There is a world of difference between knowing what to do,
and actually doing it.*
—Bill Phillips

Congratulations. You made it. You managed to read this book in its entirety, from start to finish. I hope you found it interesting, enlightening, and a little thought-provoking. Most importantly, I hope it's created an awareness that inspires you to commit to taking better care of yourself whilst working 24/7.

That commitment means you're prepared to do whatever it takes to rewrite your shift-working story, which for some of you may mean doing things a little differently, especially if your health and relationships are not where you'd like them to be right now.

Ultimately, my biggest wish is that you don't let this become one of those books that you read and talk about with your friends (although that would be lovely, thank you), only to place it on the bookshelf right next to all of your other books, without doing anything differently.

It was never written to be a passive read, a book that provides you with lots of knowledge, information, tips, and tricks, but doesn't inspire you to do things differently.

Because nothing changes, if nothing changes.

And that's not what I want for you right now.

Its why I've summarised all of the Healthy Shift Worker Actions Steps that I mentioned throughout this book, and included them, along with a handful of recipes, at the end of this book to help get you started.

All you need to do now is choose one thing from that list and begin to apply it to your shift-working life, starting today.

The word *apply* being key.

Because acquiring knowledge makes you smarter, but it doesn't make you healthier.

That requires action.

If you don't take action or change your behaviour, then things are going to stay the same (or, more likely, get worse).

So it's time to do your part and put what you've learned into action, whether that's implementing relaxation techniques to help enhance your mind and body to initiate sleep, as opposed to sedating it; reducing your food intake when working overnight which includes consuming more liquid nutrition to support digestive health; or committing to working on a relationship that has become a little strained over the years.

Whatever you choose to do, start by choosing one thing from the Healthy Shift Worker Checklist that you can begin to implement into your shift-working lifestyle that is going to make the biggest difference in your life.

Once you've mastered that one thing, choose another, and so on.

It all begins by making different choices and taking different actions, slowly and steadily, one step at a time, until they become the new norm in your life.

And don't stop there.

Be the change that you'd like to see in your workplace: a Healthy Shift Worker Ambassador of sorts. That way, you're helping your workmates to become healthy by creating a healthy shift-worker ripple effect with all those around you.

As Martin Luther King Jr so beautifully said. "Take the first step in faith. You don't have to see the whole staircase; just take the first step."

Audra x

Healthy Shift Worker Checklist

Action Steps to Help You to Work (and Survive) in a 24/7 World

Struggle 1. Ongoing and relentless sleep deprivation and disruption

Tip 1: Prioritise your sleep, no matter what.
Tip 2: Boot your phone out of the bedroom.
Tip 3: Focus on relaxation, not sedation.

Struggle 2. My uniform must be shrinking; weight fluctuations and an expanding waistline

Tip 1: Eat minimally when your digestive system is sleeping.
Tip 2: Curb the sugar cravings with healthy fats and protein.
Tip 3: Quench your thirst with water, not sugar.

Struggle 3. Feelings of stress, anxiety, and depression

Tip 1: Start going into work in an imaginary bubble.
Tip 2: Embrace the concept of saying no.
Tip 3: Go easy on the "cups of stress": coffee and energy drinks.
Tip 4: Do more of what makes you happy.
Tip 5: Increase your intake of stress-busting nutrients and food.
Tip 6: Move more regularly, but gently.
Bonus tip: Ask for help.

Struggle 4. A depleted and burnt-out immune system

Tip 1: Prioritise your sleep; take two.
Tip 2: Nourish the gut by eating more veggies.

Tip 3: Boost lymphatic flow through exercise, harnessing the benefits of rebounding.

Struggle 5. A disrupted family and social life, strained relationships, and tension in the workplace

Tip 1: Read the book *The 5 Love Languages.*
Tip 2: Set socialisation goals to connect, device free.
Tip 3: Would you like to work with you?
Bonus tip: Give a copy of this book to your friends, family, and work colleagues.

Part 5.
Healthy Shift Worker Recipes

Energising Early Shift Recipes

NOW WHEN IT comes to taking something into work for breakfast, it's easy to pack the cereal, milk, and maybe a piece of fruit into our workbag, and 'voila' we're done! The trouble with this breakfast-out-of-a-box approach is that it's made up predominantly of refined carbohydrates and sugar which means not only is it not providing your body with any form of nourishment but most notably, it's going to leave you feeling hungry about 1 hour later.

And we all know what happens next.

Bring me that coffee and muffin – stat!

It's this continual roller-coaster ride of blood sugar crashes that over time, sets us up for a whole host of chronic health conditions including insulin resistance, pre-diabetes and eventually Type 2 Diabetes. Health conditions which, unfortunately, are becoming more and more prevalent amongst those who work 24/7.

So to provide you with some nourishment and sustained energy to help power you through your early shift (without the need for copious amounts of coffee and doughnuts), it's as simple as adding more protein and healthy fats into your morning ritual.

Here's a few options to get you started:

Creamy Nut Butter Chia Puddings

(Serves 2-3)

What's great about them?

- Chia seeds and nut butter are packed full of protein and healthy omega-3 fats, so they're going to leave you feeling sustained for much longer than a bowl of cereal and toast. You can also make a batch of these in advance, and they're perfect for transporting into work in a jar.

Ingredients

- 2 cups of milk of choice (almond, coconut)
- ½ cup chia seeds
- 1 banana
- ¼ cup nut butter (almond, cashews, brazil nut)
- 4 Medjool dates, pitted and chopped
- 1 teaspoon pure vanilla extra or paste
- Toppings to serve – walnuts, pecans, flaked coconut, cacao nibs, banana, peaches, cinnamon, nutmeg etc.

How to make them!

Place milk, chia seeds and banana into a blender, and blend for 5-10 seconds. Add in the nut butter, dates and vanilla and blend until smooth by starting slowly, then gradually increasing the speed until the dates are broken down finely.

Pour into sealed jars and top with topping of choice for some added crunch and flavour. Leave in the fridge for 4 hours, or overnight.

Throw them into your workbag as you walk out the door for your early shift, and you've got yourself a delicious, filling breakfast that will keep you sustained for hours!

Ridiculously Easy Overnight Oats!

(Serves 1)

What's great about them?

- The name says it all. These overnight oats are super quick and easy to make - it's ridiculous, but in a good way!
- Adding in the Greek yoghurt and seeds boosts the protein and healthy fats which will help to keep you feeling fuller for longer, and less dependent on sugary treats and beverages.

Ingredients

- 1/3 cup of milk of choice (almond, coconut, rice)
- 1/3 cup of Greek yoghurt
- 1/3 cup of rolled oats
- 1 tablespoon raw honey
- 2 tablespoons mixed seeds (sunflower, pumpkin, chia)
- 1 teaspoon vanilla paste
- 1/3 cup frozen berries

How to make them!

Combine all of the ingredients (except for the berries), into a jar and mix well. Top with frozen berries and leave overnight in the fridge.

These are also great for when returning home from night shift, as all you need to do is remove them from the fridge when you get home and enjoy!

Note: you can double the ingredients to make a few jars in advance.

Candice's Breakfast Loaf [1]
(Serves 8-10)

(GF, Dairy Free, Refined Sugar-Free, Vegetarian, Vegan)

This recipe is from one of my nursing friends, Candice Bauer, who along with her husband Matt, are the Founders of BAREByBauer, a natural body and skincare company based here in Australia. Candice makes this delicious loaf to take into her early shift to help keep her sustained through those busy shifts in the hospital!

The prep-time for this recipe is super quick (only 10 minutes), while the cooking time is 45-60 minutes, making it a perfect meal to prepare in advance that will provide you with several breakfast options to last you through the week.

What's great about it?

- This quick'n'easy recipe is perfect to have cooked and ready to go in the fridge or freezer for a filling, nutritious breakfast.
- Oats, walnuts and coconut oil help to keep you full with healthy fats, carbohydrates and protein, whilst the bananas and berries offer sweetness and antioxidants.
- Cinnamon and ginger give it that little extra something whilst helping to stabilise blood sugar levels and promoting proper digestion.
- The zucchini ... well like I also mentioned in Chapter 4, Candice loves adding veggies and greens wherever she can because they're SO good for our overall health.

Ingredients

- 3 cups organic gluten-free oats
- 1tsp cinnamon
- 1/2tsp ground ginger
- 3-5 bananas (depending on size)

- 2-3 apples (depending on size)
- 1 medium to large zucchini
- 3tbs extra virgin coconut oil
- 1 cup walnuts
- 1 cup berries of choice (fresh or frozen)

How to make it!

1. Pre-heat oven to 180 degrees Celsius and prepare loaf tray.
2. Place oats, cinnamon and ground ginger in blended and blitz until relatively fine.
3. Add bananas and coconut oil. Blitz until smooth.
4. Add chopped apples and zucchini. Blitz until desired texture. Some like it smooth, some like it chunky.
5. Add walnuts and blitz very briefly to chop nuts (leave some chunks and crunchy nuts are delicious!)
6. Stir through berries and transfer into prepared loaf tray.
7. Cook on approximately 180 degrees Celsius for 45-60 minutes depending on oven.
8. Allow to cool and chop up into slices. Store in fridge or freezer.

Tips:

- Best served toasted or warm with a big dollop of grass-fed butter!
- Double the recipe and make 2 batches while you're going ... it saves so much time and stores incredibly well.
- Adjust cinnamon and ginger amounts to suit tastebuds or even add in some chai spices. Get creative ☺

Nourishing Night Shift Recipes

As our digestive system functions naturally slow right down during the night, we need to be mindful of what (and when) we're eating to help reduce digestive distress and gastrointestinal discomfort. These warming, nourishing and 'liquid nutrition' type meals will help to do just that.

Stewed Apple and Ginger Puddings

What's great about them?

- Stewed apples contain pectin, a type of soluble fibre which has a mild laxative effect, so can help to relieve constipation, along with reducing that uncomfortable feeling of bloating. It can also contribute to firm stools and reduce inflammation associated with diarrhea.
- Pectin acts as a prebiotic, in that it increases the short-chain fatty acid butyrate that feeds the beneficial micro-organisms in the gut while decreasing the population of harmful bacteria.
- Ginger can help to settle an upset stomach and reduce nausea, which is common in many night shift workers.
- Kefir is a fermented drink made from cultures of yeast and lactic acid bacteria high in nutrients and probiotics and has potent antibacterial properties which can help protect against infections.

Ingredients

- 6 organic apples
- 1/2 cup filtered water
- 1/2 cup sultanas (for added sweetness and fibre)
- 2cm piece of ginger, grated
- 2 teaspoons cinnamon (helps with blood sugar regulation)
- 1/2 cup of kefir or yoghurt to serve

How to make them?

Peel and core the apples and chop them into small evenly sized pieces. Put all the ingredients (except the kefir or yoghurt), in a covered pan and cook for about 15 minutes, stirring regularly. Cook until the pieces are soft and the colour turns light brown from the cinnamon.

Pop small batches of the pudding into small containers (the equivalent of about 1 apple each), which can be transported into work, and then leave in the fridge until ready to eat.

For an added gut-healing effect, drizzle with goat's milk kefir.

Sprinkle with cinnamon – helps to stabilise blood sugar.

Roasted Pear, Onion and Beetroot Soup [2]
(Serves 4)

I've tweaked and adapted this recipe from Christine Bailey's 'Spiced Roasted Beetroot & Apple Soup' which features in her book – *The Gut Health Diet Plan**. Christine's book contains loads of delicious gut-nourishing recipes that are designed to restore digestive health, along with giving our health and wellbeing a bit of a boost – which is exactly what a tired and weary shift worker needs, especially on night shifts.

What's great about it?

- This soup is a great pick-me-up alternative to coffee or any other caffeinated beverage as beetroots are abundant in dietary nitrates. When the body breaks down nitrates into nitric oxide, it increases oxygen flow to the brain, thereby enhancing mental clarity and alertness.
- Onions contain chromium, which helps to stabilise blood sugar, and the pears add a natural sweetness to this dish.
- Fennel seeds and ginger can also help to settle an upset stomach – 'night shift nausea' being prevalent in those working during the night.

Ingredients

- 500g beetroot, peeled and diced
- 2 pears, cored and cut into quarters
- 2 peeled garlic cloves, whole
- 4 shallot onions, cut in half
- 1 cm fresh ginger, finely grated
- 3 tbsp olive oil

- 1 tsp fennel seeds
- 1 tsp cumin seeds
- ½ tsp ground coriander
- 1-litre chicken or beef stock/broth
- Zest and juice of 2 limes
- Small bunch mint leaves, finely chopped
- 200g Greek yoghurt or kefir to serve

How to make it!

Preheat oven to 180degrees Celsius, then place the chopped beetroot, pears, onion and garlic into a bowl. Drizzle the oil over the top and mix well - transfer to a roasting pan, and roast for 50 minutes or until soft.

Place the fennel and cumin seeds in a pan, and dry roast over medium heat for about 1 minute. Combine the roasted vegetables with the fennel and cumin seeds, along with the remaining ingredients (excluding the mint and yoghurt). Add to a food processor and puree until the soup has a smooth texture.

Heat in a saucepan over medium heat for approximately 5 minutes, then pour into a thermos or hot flask to take into work. To serve, dollop a spoonful of yoghurt or kefir over the soup, then top with a sprinkle of mint.

* Recipe adapted and reproduced with permission of the Licensor through PLSclear.

Nourishing Coconut, Lime and Blueberry Night Shift Jellies

What's great about them?

- These are great 'comfort food' alternatives to those bags of lollies or cakes that we often bring into work for the night shift!
- Gelatin is made up of 98-99% protein and has been shown to improve brain function and memory, as well as the appearance of skin, hair and nails.
- Nourishing on the gut as gelatin contains the amino acid, glutamic acid, which is converted to glutamine in the body. Glutamine has been shown to improve the integrity of the gut lining and help in the prevention of "leaky gut".
- Blueberries are low in carbohydrates, loaded with antioxidants and contain multiple anti-inflammatory properties to reduce inflammation.

Ingredients

- ¼ cup Changing Habits Gelatin Powder
- 100ml Coconut Milk
- 1 teaspoon of Vanilla Bean Paste
- 200g frozen blueberries
- 1 lime, juiced
- 1 tablespoon of Organic Honey or pure Maple Syrup

How to make them!

Blend the lime and blueberries in a food processor until thoroughly mixed.

Pour the mixture into a saucepan. Add the vanilla, honey and gelatin and whisk together. Warm the ingredients on low heat until the gelatin dissolves, stirring continuously, but not letting it boil.

Remove from the heat and whisk in the coconut milk. Pour into moulds and place in the fridge for a least 1 hour until firm.

Slow Cooked Chicken and Corn Chowder with Gremolata [3]

This simple, delicious and nutritious recipe is from a fellow nutritionist, Mary-Leigh Scheerhoorn, who I went to University with, and had lots of things in common. Going back to "school" in our 40's was one of them!

This recipe makes up over a litre of chowder so there is enough to eat for a few meals. It will keep in the fridge for 2 - 3 days or you can portion it up and pop it in the freezer for a quick go-to meal when you're short on time. Warm dishes are great to have through the night, especially when our body temperature naturally drops around 2-4am, or to have just before jumping into bed after night shift.

What's great about it?

- Garlic contains antibacterial, antiviral and anti-fungal compounds which help to support the immune system.
- The protein in the chicken and stock contains glutamine, an essential amino acid which helps to reduce inflammation, support the integrity of the intestinal wall, and enable the body to heal and nourish itself.
- Slow cooking ingredients allow the foods to be broken down into more easily digestible pieces, thereby minimising digestive distress and discomfort.

Ingredients

- 1-2 glugs of extra virgin olive oil
- 1 large brown onion – peeled and finely diced
- 2 medium carrots – washed and finely diced
- 2 ribs of celery – washed and finely diced

- 1-2 cloves of garlic – peeled and finely diced or minced
- 1 tbsp chopped thyme (or lemon thyme)
- 3-4 medium potatoes – washed, skin on, diced – about 1cm square (roughly)
- 2 cobs of corn – remove the kernels by cutting down the side of the corn cob (or use 1 cup of frozen corn kernels)
- 1-litre good quality chicken stock (low sodium – add your own salt at the end)
- 2 chicken Marylands – (thigh/leg on the bone)
- 2-3 bay leaves
- 1/2 cup cream (optional)
- 1 can white beans - rinsed and drained (optional)
- Salt and pepper to taste

The Gremolata

1 lemon - zest only
2 tbsp parsley - chopped
1 clove garlic - minced
1 tsp olive oil

How to make it!

Slow cooker with sauté function*

1. Gently sauté the onion, carrot and celery for about 5 minutes or until the onion has gone translucent.
2. Add garlic and thyme and sauté for another couple of minutes before adding in the potatoes, corn kernels and chicken stock.
3. Place the chicken into the slow cooker, seal the lid and set to 8 hours/overnight.
4. When the timer is finished, gently remove the chicken Marylands and bay leaves.
5. Skim off any scum that might have come to the surface of the soup/stock.
6. Remove the meat off the chicken, discarding the skin, bone and gristle.
7. Shred the chicken and put aside.
8. Use a stick blender to blend the vegetables. If using the white beans, you can add them in now (they will add to the thickness of the chowder and give a nourishing fibre and protein boost).
9. Add the shredded chicken and cream (if you choose that option).
10. To make the gremolata - mix the lemon zest, parsley, garlic and olive oil into a paste-like consistency. You can add a bit of lemon juice and salt and pepper if you like.
11. Serve the chowder with a sprinkling of gremolata and some crusty sourdough bread.

*The sautéing of the vegetables helps to release their sweetness and adds an extra depth to the flavour, however, the chowder will still taste good if you miss this step because you don't have time before leaving for your shift or the energy before falling into bed!

Curb Sugar-Cravings

When we're running on little sleep, our sugar-cravings can go into overdrive because our body is instinctively seeking out energy that it's not getting from a restorative night's rest.

And the fastest, most accessible source of energy that our body can use is, you guessed it – sugar! Or more scientifically, glucose, which means if you don't get sufficient sleep, you're going to have some serious carbohydrate cravings.

So what can we do about it besides getting more sleep? Adding more protein and healthy fats into your diet will help to reduce those blood glucose spikes, along with including snacks that are going to help to sustain you, and keep you feeling fuller for longer. Here are a few to get you inspired!

Lara's Spiced Pumpkin Hummus [4]

I first met Lara Busch back in 2010, in a pathophysiology class when we were still nutrition students, and always admired her keen interest in mental health.

Research has undeniably shown a strong correlation between our mental health and the nutrients that we're getting (or not getting) from the food that we eat. This is because our gut bugs or microbiome rely heavily on a diversified diet of plant foods so that they can produce important neurotransmitters that help to boost our mood. It's why I love Lara's take on the traditional hummus recipe, as she's added some pumpkin along with sesame seeds that are rich in micronutrients such as copper, iron, zinc and magnesium to boost brain function.

What's great about it?

- Hummus originates in the Middle East and is often consumed in a mezza-style platter.
- Traditionally it contains chickpeas, garlic, lemon and tahini, but this has a different twist.
- It's also a filling snack to have with some vegetable sticks, or alongside a main meal as it's a great source of complex carbohydrates and protein.

Ingredients

- 1 cup pumpkin, diced
- 2 tsp sesame seeds
- 400g tin chickpeas, rinsed
- 2 cloves garlic, finely chopped
- 2 tsp extra virgin olive oil

- ½ lemon, freshly squeezed
- ½ cup parsley, fined chopped
- ½- 1 tsp curry powder (to taste)
- Salt (to taste)

How to make it!

Season pumpkin with salt and coat in 1 tsp olive oil. Roast pumpkin in the oven on 180 degrees, for 25 minutes.

Blend all the ingredients in a food processor or high- speed blender, until a smooth consistency.

Serve the dip with capsicum, carrot, cucumber, snow pea crudites and seed crackers or whatever is desired.

Walnut, Prune and Cinnamon Logs
(Makes 10-12)

What's great about them?

Walnuts are high in antioxidants and omega-3 fatty acids which are great for brain function and cognition.

- Prunes are full of fibre and taste very sweet, so can be a healthy alternative to satisfying sugar cravings which occur when we haven't had enough sleep.
- Prunes also contain sorbitol, a naturally occurring sugar alcohol that is absorbed slowly in the digestive gut, thereby minimising blood sugar spikes.

Ingredients

- 1 ½ cups prunes (dried plums)
- 1 cup walnuts or pecans
- 1 tablespoon chia seeds
- 2 tablespoons coconut oil
- 1 dessert spoon cinnamon
- 1 teaspoon vanilla paste
- ½ cup desiccated coconut (topping)

How to make them!

Place all the ingredients into a food processor except the coconut, and combine until everything is blended well. Roll a tablespoon of the mixture into log shapes, and finish by rolling in coconut.

Bring into work to share with your workmates!

Sara's Caprese Skewers [5]

These tasty but straightforward savoury snacks are from my friend Sara Capacci, who is originally from Cesena in Italy and is an absolute whiz in the kitchen. According to Sara, in Italy, Caprese is offered in restaurants as an entrée (antipasto) only when tomatoes are in season, so it's unlikely to find Caprese in other seasons. When combined, the colours also represent the Italian flag: the basil is green, the Bocconcini Mozzarella is white and the tomatoes red.

While the Italians may use it as an appetiser, I think it's versatility makes them great for sharing around the workplace on night shift!

What's great about them?

- Tomatoes are made up of 95% water, so are a great way to sneak in a bit of extra hydration, which is a signficant contributor to fatigue. Although they're technically a fruit, their carbohydrate content is minimal (just 5% including fibre), so they're not going to spike your blood sugar levels.
- Tomatoes are also high in many vitamins and minerals (vitamins C and K, potassium and folate), along with *lycopene*, an antioxidant linked to many health benefits including heart health and certain types of cancers.
- Basil has both anti-bacterial and anti-inflammatory qualities, and Mozarella is a soft, white cheese that is not only filling, but also contains probiotics that may help to boost your immune system.

Ingredients

- 200g Cherry Tomatoes (preferably spray free or organic)
- 200g Bocconcini Mozzarella cheese
- Few basil leaves

How to make it!

Wash tomatoes and basil leaves.

Cut tomatoes in halves and do the same with the Bocconcini.

Make a skewer using a toothpick and combining half Mozzarella, the basil leaf and the half tomato.

Place them on a serving plate to bring into work to share with your workmates, and season with salt, pepper & extra virgin olive oil.

Organic Medjool Dates Stuffed With Nut Butter
(Serves 1)

What's great about them?

- Dates are great natural sweeteners designed by Mother Nature that provide a natural pick-me-up to help ward off fatigue and tiredness, in particular when experiencing those sugar cravings at 3am.
- They are high in soluble fibre which helps to alleviate constipation by keeping bowel movements regular.
- Nut butters are high in plant-based fats and protein, and studies have shown walnuts can help to improve brain function.

Ingredients

- 2 Medjool dates
- 2 teaspoons of nut butter (almond, cashew, brazil nut)
- 2 walnuts

How to make them!

Slice open each date (avoid cutting them in half completely) and remove the pits.

Add a teaspoon of nut butter to each date, then top with a walnut.

Enjoy with a cuppa at 3am, or whenever you start feeling the onset of sugar cravings.

Greek Yoghurt with Cinnamon, Chia and Berries

(Serves 1)

What's great about them?

- Greek yoghurt is much thicker and creamier than regular yoghurt, and also much higher in protein which is going to keep you feeling fuller for longer. It's especially helpful for those trying to lose weight.
- Fresh berries are naturally sweet which will help to satisfy the sugar cravings, along with being full of fibre, vitamins and minerals.
- Cinnamon helps to improve insulin sensitivity thereby reducing insulin resistance, a condition quite prevalent in those working 24/7.
- Chia seeds also help to reduce insulin resistance and improve blood sugar control.

Ingredients

- 4 heaped tablespoons of Greek yoghurt
- A handful of berries (or seasonal fruit of choice)
- 1/4 teaspoon cinnamon
- 1 teaspoon chia seeds

How to make it!

Place yoghurt into a small jar with a leak proof lid and add berries. Sprinkle cinnamon and chia seeds over the top. Tighten the lid and take into work to enjoy whenever those sugar cravings turn into over-drive!

Note: Coconut Yoghurt or Kefir made from coconut milk are great dairy-free options that are packed with gut nourishing probiotics.

Special Thanks

In all honesty, this book would not have come to fruition had it not been for one incredible human being: Marcus Pearce, CEO of the Wellness Couch podcast network. Thanks to his constant encouragement and belief in my healthy shift-worker message, *The Healthy Shift Worker Podcast* first graced the airwaves back in February 2016. Having also read earlier versions of my manuscript over the years, along with sending gentle reminders of "Audra, you really need to get that book finished because shift workers need to read it," I definitely owe your ongoing support for *Too Tired to Cook* coming to life.

Tanya Outridge, for sewing-the-seed in my mind so many years ago to embark on a career where I work solely with shift workers. It was such a defining moment as it made me realise my true purpose in life. To collectively empower shift workers to take better care of their health, in order to help them to transition from unhealthy to healthy.

To Cyndi O'Meara, for writing the foreword, and for being one of the biggest influencers in improving my health over the years, and eventual career change to becoming a nutritionist myself. I picked up your book *Changing Habits, Changing Lives* when you first wrote it in the 1990s, and wow, what an eye-opening read that was (and still is). I've pretty much been following you ever since, including graduating from your Functional Nutrition Academy, as I continue to learn from you every single day.

To Tracey Rohweder, for also writing the foreword, and for being my self-proclaimed #number1hswfan. It was an easy decision for me to ask you to co-write the foreword, as you've played such an integral role in helping me spread the healthy shift-worker message to a much larger audience. Not to mention you were brave enough to come in and see me while I was still on my "L" plates, studying to become a nutritionist, and hung around to become good friends ever since. I also love that you're a Roger Federer fan too, so I knew we were destined to be friends for life!

To Candice, Sara, Lara, and Mary-Leigh for contributing recipes to this book. I've really enjoyed taste-testing your recipes, and I'm sure our readers are going to love them just as much as I do.

To all of my friends (you know who you are) who have had my back and been everlasting with your support of constant encouragement in my quest to help shift workers around the globe. Changing careers in your forties is incredibly scary, and I'm happy to admit there were plenty of times when I was gripped with self-doubt and asked myself whether I'm doing the right thing with my life. So suffice to say, I could not have made this journey without you.

These people include my Exceptional Life Blueprint friends; we met through Marcus Pearce: Alison, Michelle, Cara, Debbie, Wendy, and Jodie. You have all gone above and beyond at getting behind my mission, and for that, I will be forever grateful.

Collette, Lara, Silvana, Sara, and Leslie-Ann, my fellow uni friends, who like me, were sitting in a pathophysiology class back in 2010 feeling like a deer in headlights. Seriously, what were we thinking?

To my former airline friends and family from Ansett and Qantas; there are too many to mention, but Kellie O'Brien, Tracie Porter, Rebecca McMaster, and Heather Drummond definitely come to mind as people who have been forever cheering me on in the background.

To my two besties, Karen and Ingrid, for twenty-plus years of friendship that all began when we started our shift working journeys together in the airline industry. Here's to endless girls lunches and catch-ups well into our nineties.

To Dale, my gorgeous shift-working husband. You have been on the receiving end of many of my healthy shift worker ideas and recipe concoctions over the years, and you're still alive to tell the tale (LOL). I'm so grateful that we met on that aerobridge all those years ago, and I love you more and more each day.

To every person who has sat in on one of my Healthy Shift Worker Workplace Wellness Seminars; I've loved meeting you face-to-face, and really appreciated your participation, feedback and being open to hear what I have to say.

The more than fifteen thousand followers of my Facebook Page (The Healthy Shift Worker) and Healthy Shift Workers Facebook Group, along with more than thirty-five thousand listeners from all around the world who have taken the time to download an episode from my podcast, thank you for all of the lovely comments and feedback. You've certainly inspired me to keep on doing what I do, knowing that I may never get to meet you in person but can help you via the written word or from a conversation on my podcast.

And finally, to all of my clients for allowing me to help you to improve your health in some way, shape, or form whilst working 24/7. You are living proof that by simply changing our mindset and behaviour, coupled together with a sheer determination to prioritise our health, it's absolutely possible to become a healthy shift worker, even when faced with many challenges.

As the late Audrey Hepburn so beautifully said, "Nothing is impossible. The word itself says I'm possible."

You just have to want it badly enough.

References

Dedication

1   Australian Bureau of Statistics 2015, *Characteristics of employment, Australia, 2015*, http://www.abs.gov.au/ausstats/abs@.nsf/Previousproducts/6333.0Main%20Features2August%202015?opendocument&tabname=Summary&prodno=6333.0&issue=August%202015&num=&view=

2   Sun, M, Feng, W, Wang, F, Li, P, Li, Z, Li, M, Tse, G, Vlaanderen, J, Vermeulen, R & Tse, L 2018, 'Meta-analysis on shift work and risks of specific obesity types', *Obesity Reviews*, vol. 19, no. 1, pp. 28-40, https://www.ncbi.nlm.nih.gov/pubmed/28975706

Ongoing and Relentless Sleep Deprivation

1   Hillman D & Lack, L 2013 'Public health implications of sleep loss: the community burden', *The Medical Journal of Australia*, vol. 199, no. 8, pp. 7-10, https://www.mja.com.au/journal/2013/199/8/public-health-implications-sleep-loss-community-burden

2   Better Health Channel 2018, *Shiftwork*, https://www.betterhealth.vic.gov.au/health/HealthyLiving/shiftwork

3   Cirelli, C & Tononi, G 2017, 'The sleeping brain', *Cerebrum*, vol. 2017, pp. 7-17, https://www.ncbi.nlm.nih.gov/pmc/articles/PMC5501041/

4   Parliament of the Commonwealth of Australia 2019, *Bedtime Reading – Inquiry into Sleep Health Awareness in Australia*, https://www.sleep.org.au/documents/item/4270?fbclid=IwAR1ia-mjuxnFxt6lMyXV3h9rhJ6yHM611SHteEolFD4V_ji6uGkFeDR5WrQ

5   National Institute of Neurological Disorders and Stroke 2018, *Brain basics: understanding sleep*, https://www.ninds.nih.gov/Disorders/Patient-Caregiver-Education/Understanding-Sleep

6   Akerstedt, T & Wright, Jr., K 2009, 'Sleep loss and fatigue in shift work and shift work disorder', *Sleep Medicine Clinics*, vol. 4, no. 2, pp. 257-271, https://www.ncbi.nlm.nih.gov/pmc/articles/PMC2904525/

7   National Sleep Foundation 2018, *What happens when you sleep?*, https://sleepfoundation.org/how-sleep-works/what-happens-when-you-sleep

8   National Sleep Foundation 2018, *Sleep Drive and Your Body Clock*, http://www.sleepfoundation.org/sleep-topics/sleep-drive-and-your-body-clock

9   Bjorness, T & Greene, R 2009, 'Adenosine and Sleep', *Current Neuropharmacology*, vol. 7, no. 3, pp. 238-245, https://www.ncbi.nlm.nih.gov/pubmed/20190965

10 Morris, C, Aeschbach, D & Scheer, F 2012, 'Circadian system, sleep and endocrinology', *Molecular and Cellular Endocrinology*, vol. 349, no. 1, pp. 91-104, https://www.ncbi.nlm.nih.gov/pubmed/21939733

11 Bulkeley K 2014, 'Why sleep deprivation is torture', *Psychology Today*, https://www.psychologytoday.com/au/blog/dreaming-in-the-digital-age/201412/why-sleep-deprivation-is-torture

12 Schwartz, T 2011, 'Sleep is more important than food', *Harvard Business Review*, https://hbr.org/2011/03/sleep-is-more-important-than-f

13 Walker, M 2017, *Why we sleep*, Penguin Random House, Great Britain.

14 Eugene, A & Masiak J 2015, 'The neuroprotective aspects of sleep', *MEDtube Science*, vol. 3, no.1, pp. 35-40, https://www.ncbi.nlm.nih.gov/pubmed/26594659

15 Shokri-Kojori, E, Wang, G, Wiers, C, Demiral, S, Guo, M, Kim, S, Lindgren, E, Ramirez, V, Zehra, A, Freeman, C, Miller, G, Manza, P, Srivastava, T, De Santi, S, Tomasi, D, Benveniste, H & Volkow, N 2018, 'β-Amyloid accumulation in the human brain after one night of sleep deprivation', *Proceedings of the National Academy of Sciences of the United States of America*, vol. 115, no. 17, pp. 4483-4488, https://www.ncbi.nlm.nih.gov/pubmed/29632177

16 Marquie, J, Tucker, P, Folkard, S, Gentil, C & Ansiau, D 2015, 'Chronic effects of shift work on cognition: findings from the VISAT longitudinal study', *Occupational & Environmental Medicine*, vol. 72, no. 4, pp. 258-264, https://oem.bmj.com/content/72/4/258

17 Xie, L, Kang, H, Xu, Q, Chen, M, Liao, Y, Thiyagarajan, M, O'Donnell, J, Christensen, D, Nicholson, C, Lliff, J, Takano, T, Deane, R & Nedergaard, M 2013, 'Sleep drives metabolite clearance from the adult brain', *Science*, vol. 342, no. 6156, pp. 373-377, https://www.ncbi.nlm.nih.gov/pubmed/24136970

18 De-Sola Gutiérrez, J, Rodríguez de Fonseca, F & Rubio, G 2016, 'Cell-phone addiction: A review', *Frontiers in Psychiatry*, vol. 7, no. 175, pp. 1-15, https://www.ncbi.nlm.nih.gov/pmc/articles/PMC5076301/

19 Archer, D 2013, 'Smartphone addiction', *Psychology Today*, https://www.psychologytoday.com/blog/reading-between-the-headlines/201307/smartphone-addiction

20 Rosekind, M, Gregory, K, Mallis, M, Brandt, S, Seal, B & Lerner, D 2010, 'The cost of poor sleep: workplace productivity loss, and associated costs', *Journal of Occupational and Environmental Medicine*, vol. 52, no. 1, pp. 91-98, https://www.ncbi.nlm.nih.gov/pubmed/20042880

21 Williamson, A & Feyer, A 2000, 'Moderate sleep deprivation produces impairments in cognitive and motor performance equivalent to legally prescribed levels of alcohol intoxication', *Occupational & Environmental Medicine*, vol. 57, no. 10, pp. 649-655, https://oem.bmj.com/content/57/10/649

22 Hampton, K, Rainie, L, Lu, W, Shin, I & Purcell, K 2015, 'Psychological stress and social media use', *Pew Research Center*, http://www.pewinternet.org/2015/01/15/psychological-stress-and-social-media-use-2/#fn-12666-9.

23   Duffy, J & Czeisler, C 2009, 'Effect on light on human circadian physiology', *Sleep Medicine Clinics*, vol. 4, no. 2, pp. 165-177, https://www.ncbi.nlm.nih.gov/pmc/articles/PMC2717723/

24   Gooley, J, Chamberlain, K, Smith, K, Khalsa, S, Rajaratnam, S, Van Reen, E, Zeitzer, J, Czeisler, C & Lockley, S 2011, 'Exposure to room light before bedtime suppresses melatonin onset and shortens melatonin duration in humans', *The Journal of Clinical Endocrinology & Metabolism*, vol. 96, no. 3, pp. 463-472, https://www.ncbi.nlm.nih.gov/pubmed/21193540

25   Chang A, Aeschbach D, Duffy J & Czeisler C 2015, 'Evening use of light-emitting eReaders negatively affects sleep, circadian timing, and next-morning alertness', *Proceedings of the National Academy of Sciences*, vol. 112, no. 4, pp. 1232-37, https://www.pnas.org/content/112/4/1232

26   Kavarana, Z, 2019, '15 Effective alarm clocks that aren't a total snooze', *Best*, https://www.bestproducts.com/appliances/small/g885/cool-alarm-clocks/

27   Arnold, L 2018, *Undrugged sleep: From insomnia to un-somnia – why sleeping pills don't improve sleep and the drug-free solutions that will*, Balboa Press, Bloomington.

28   Garber, S 2013, 'The difference between natural and chemically-induced sleep', *HuffPost*, https://www.huffpost.com/entry/natural-chemical-sleep_b_3743923

29   Harvard Health Publications 2015, *Relaxation techniques: Breath control helps quell errant stress response*, http://www.health.harvard.edu/mind-and-mood/relaxation-techniques-breath-control-helps-quell-errant-stress-response.

30   Weill, A 2015, *Asleep in 60 seconds: 4-7-8 breathing technique claims to help you to nod off in just a minute*, https://www.youtube.com/watch?v=gz4G31LGyog&t=3s

31   St-Onge, M, Roberts, A, Shechter, A & Choudhury, A 2016, 'Fiber and saturated fat are associated with sleep arousals and slow wave sleep', *Journal of Clinical Sleep Medicine*, vol. 12, no. 1, pp. 19-24, https://www.ncbi.nlm.nih.gov/pubmed/26156950

32   Cao, Y, Wittert, G, Taylor, A, Adams, R & Shi, Z 2016, 'Associations between macronutrient intake and obstructive sleep apnoea as well as self-reported sleep

symptoms: Results from a cohort of community dwelling Australian Men', *Nutrients*, vol. 8, no. 4, pp. 1-14, https://www.mdpi.com/2072-6643/8/4/207

33   Kohsaka, A, Laposky, A, Ramsey, K, Estrada, C, Joshu, C, Kobayashi, Y, Turek, F & Bass, J 2007, 'High-fat diet disrupts behavioral and molecular circadian rhythms in mice', *Cell Metabolism*, vol. 6, no. 5, pp. 414-421, https://www.ncbi.nlm.nih.gov/pubmed/17983587

34   Fereidoun, H & Pouria, H 2014, 'Effect of excessive salt consumption on night's sleep', *Pakistan Journal of Physiology*, vol. 10, no. 3-4, pp. 6-9, http://www.pps.org.pk/PJP/10-3/Hyderpour.pdf

Weight Fluctuations and an Expanding Waistline

1   Greer, S, Goldstein, A & Walker, M 2013, 'The impact of sleep deprivation on food desire in the human brain', *Nature Communications*, vol. 4, no. 2259, pp. 1-19, https://www.ncbi.nlm.nih.gov/pubmed/23922121

2   School of Medicine and Public Health 2013, 'How the tired brain directs junk-food binges', *University of Wisconsin-Madison*, http://www.med.wisc.edu/news-events/how-the-tired-brain-directs-junk-food-binges/41439

3   Van Cauter, E, Spiegel, K, Tasali, E & Leproult, R 2008, 'Metabolic consequences of sleep and sleep loss, *Sleep Medicine*, vol. 9, no. 1, pp. 23-28, https://www.ncbi.nlm.nih.gov/pmc/articles/PMC4444051/

4   Hogenkamp, P, Nilsson, E, Nilsson, V, Chapman, C, Vogel, H, Lundberg, L, Zarei, S, Cedernaes, J, Rangtell, F, Broman, J, Dickson, S, Brunstrom, J, Benedict, C, & Schioth, H 2013, 'Acute sleep deprivation increases portion size and affects food choice in young men', *Psychoneuroendocrinology*, vol. 38, no. 9, pp. 1668-1674, https://www.ncbi.nlm.nih.gov/pubmed/23428257

5   National Sleep Foundation 2017, *Lack of sleep may increase calorie consumption*, https://sleepfoundation.org/sleep-news/lack-sleep-may-increase-calorie-consumption

6   Jackson, S, Kirschbaum, C & Steptoe, A 2017, 'Hair cortisol and adiposity in a population-based sample of 2,527 men and women aged 54 to 87 years', *Obesity*, vol. 25, no. 3, pp. 539-544, https://www.ncbi.nlm.nih.gov/pubmed/28229550

7   Godman, H 2012, 'Losing weight and belly fat improves sleep', *Harvard Health Publications*, http://www.health.harvard.edu/blog/losing-weight-and-belly-fat-improves-sleep-201211145531

8   Spaeth, A, Dinges, D & Goel, N 2013, 'Effects of experimental sleep restriction on weight gain, caloric intake, and meal timing in healthy adults', *Sleep*, vol. 36, no. 7, pp. 981-990, https://www.ncbi.nlm.nih.gov/pubmed/23814334

9   Spiegel, K, Tasali, E, Penev, P & Van Cauter, E 2004, 'Sleep curtailment in healthy young men is associated with decreased leptin levels, elevated ghrelin levels, and increased hunger and appetite', *Annals of Internal Medicine*, vol. 141, no. 11, pp. 846-850, https://www.ncbi.nlm.nih.gov/pubmed/15583226

10   Rind, B 2009, 'Treating Low Metabolism', *Wise Traditions In Food, Farming and The Healing Arts*, vol. 10, no. 2, pp. 1-128, https://www.westonaprice.org/wp-content/uploads/Summer2009.pdf

11   Weaver, L 2011, *Accidentally Overweight*, Allen & Unwin, St Leonards.

12   Bravo R, Ugartemendia L, Uguz C, Rodríguez A & Cubero J 2017, 'Current opinions in chrononutrition and health', *Journal of Clinical Nutrition and Dietetics*, vol. 3, no. 1, pp. 1-3, http://clinical-nutrition.imedpub.com/current-opinions-in-chrononutrition-and-health.pdf

13   Almoosawi, S, Vingeliene, S, Gachon, F, Voortman, T, Palla, L, Johnston, J, Martinus Van Dam, R, Darimont, C & Karagounis, L 2018, 'Chronotype: Implications for epidemiologic studies on chrono-nutrition and cardiometabolic health', *Advances in Nutrition*, vol. 10, no.1, pp. 30-42, https://www.ncbi.nlm.nih.gov/pubmed/30500869

14   Pot, G, Almoosawi, S & Stephen, A 2016, 'Meal irregularity and cardiometabolic consequences: results from observational and intervention studies', *Proceedings of the Nutrition Society*, vol. 75, no. 4, pp. 475-486, https://www.ncbi.nlm.nih.gov/pubmed/27327128

15   Asher, G & Sassone-Corsi, P 2015, 'Time for food: the interplay between nutrition, metabolism and the circadian clock', *Cell*, vol. 161, no. 1, pp. 84-92, https://www.ncbi.nlm.nih.gov/pubmed/25815987

16 Arble, D, Bass, J, Laposky, A, Vitaternal, M & Turek, F 2009, 'Circadian timing of food intake contributes to weight gain', *Obesity (Silver Spring)*, vol. 17, no. 11, pp. 2100-2102, https://www.ncbi.nlm.nih.gov/pubmed/19730426

17 Escobar, C, Angeles-Castellanos, M, Noemi, E, Bautista, R & Buijs, R 2016, 'Food during the night is the leading cause of obesity', *Mexican Journal of Eating Disorders*, vol. 7, no. 1, pp. 78-83, https://www.sciencedirect.com/science/article/pii/S2007152316000045

18 Almoosawi, S, Vingeliene, S, Karagounis, L & Pot, G 2016, 'Chrono-nutrition: a review of current evidence from observational studies on global trends in time-of-day of energy intake and its association with obesity', *Proceedings of the Nutrition Society*, vol. 75, no. 4, pp. 487-500, https://www.ncbi.nlm.nih.gov/pubmed/27327252

19 Vaughn, B, Rotolo, S & Roth H 2014, 'Circadian Rhythms and Sleep Influences on Digestive Physiology and Disorders', *ChronoPhysiology and Therapy*, vol. 4, pp. 67-77, https://www.researchgate.net/publication/274276764_Circadian_rhythm_and_sleep_influences_on_digestive_physiology_and_disorders

20 Morris, C, Yang, J, Garcia, J, Myers, S, Bozzi, I, Wang, W, Buxton, O, Shea, S & Scheer, F 2015, 'Endogenous circadian system and circadian misalignment impact glucose tolerance via separate mechanisms in humans', *Proceedings of the National Academy of Sciences*, pp. 2225-2234, https://www.pnas.org/content/112/17/E2225

21 Salgado-Delgado, R, Angeles-Castellanos, M, Saderi, N, Buijs, R & Escobar, C 2010, 'Food intake during the normal activity phase prevents obesity and circadian desynchrony in a rat model of night work', *Endocrinology*, vol. 151, no. 3, pp. 1019-1029, https://www.ncbi.nlm.nih.gov/pubmed/20080873

22 Jiang, P & Turek, F 2017, 'Timing of meals: When is as critical as what and how much', *American Journal of Physiology, Endocrinology & Metabolism*, vol. 312, no. 5, pp. 369-380, https://www.ncbi.nlm.nih.gov/pmc/articles/PMC6105931/

23 Panda, S & Gill S 2015, ' A Smartphone App reveals erratic diurnal eating patterns in humans that can be modulated for health benefits', *Cell Metabolism*, vol. 22, no. 5, pp. 789-798, https://www.cell.com/cell-metabolism/fulltext/S1550-4131(15)00462-3

24 Campbell-McBride, N 2010, *Gut and psychology syndrome*, Medinform Publishing, United Kingdom.

25 West, H 2017, *18 Healthy Foods To Eat When Cravings Strike*, Authority Nutrition, https://www.healthline.com/nutrition/18-healthy-foods-cravings

26 Palsdottir, H 2016, *15 Foods That Are Incredibly Filling*, Authority Nutrition, https://www.healthline.com/nutrition/15-incredibly-filling-foods

27 Gunnars, K 2017, *12 Proven Health Benefits of Avocado*, Authority Nutrition, https://www.healthline.com/nutrition/12-proven-benefits-of-avocado #section1

28 Fowler, S, Williams, K, Hazuda, H 2015, 'Diet soda intake is associated with long-term increases in waist circumference in a biethnic cohort of older adults: The San Antonia longitudinal study of aging', *Journal of the American Geriatrics Society*, vol. 63, no. 4, pp. 708-715, https://www.ncbi.nlm.nih.gov/ pubmed/25780952

29 Chen, L, Appel, L, Loria, C, Lin, P, Champagne, C, Elmer, P, Ard, J, Mitchell, D, Batch, B, Svetkey, L & Caballero, B 2009, 'Reduction in consumption of sugar-sweetened beverages is associated with weight loss: the PREMIER trial', *The American Journal of Clinical Nutrition*, vol. 89, no. 5, pp. 1299-1306, https://www.ncbi.nlm.nih.gov/pubmed/19339405

Feelings of Stress, Anxiety and Depression

1 Naviaux, R 2014, 'Metabolic features of the cell danger response', *Mitochondrion*, vol. 16, pp. 7-17, https://www.sciencedirect.com/science/ article/pii/S1567724913002390

2 Singh, K 2016, 'Nutrient and Stress Management', *Journal of Nutrition & Food Sciences*, vol. 6, no. 4, pp. 1-6, https://www.omicsonline.org/open-access/nutrient -and-stress-management-2155-9600-1000528.pdf

3 Tsigos, C & Chrousos, G 2002, 'Hypothalamic-pituitary-adrenal axis, neuroendocrine factors and stress', *Journal of Psychosomatic Research*, vol. 53, no. 4, pp. 865-871, https://www.ncbi.nlm.nih.gov/pubmed/12377295

4   Harvard Health Publishing 2010, *Taking aim at belly fat*, https://www.health.harvard.edu/staying-healthy/taking-aim-at-belly-fat

5   Rulanda, L, van Kruysbergen, G, de Jong, F, Koper, J & van Rossum, E 2011, 'Shift work at young age is associated with elevated long-term cortisol levels and body mass index', *The Journal of Clinical Endocrinology & Metabolism*, vol. 96, no. 11, pp. 1862-1885, https://www.ncbi.nlm.nih.gov/pubmed/21880805

6   Foster, R 2013, *Why do we sleep?*, Ted Global, https://www.ted.com/talks/russell_foster_why_do_we_sleep

7   Wang, S & Wu, W 2005, 'Effects of psychological stress on small intestinal motility and bacteria and mucosa in mice', *World Journal of Gastroenterology*, vol. 11, no. 3, pp. 2016-2021, https://www.ncbi.nlm.nih.gov/pubmed/15800998

8   Sookoian, S, Gemma, C, Gianotti, T, Burgueno, A, Alvarez, A, Gonzalez, C & Pirola, C 2007, 'Serotonin and serotonin transporter gene variant in rotating shift workers', *SLEEP*, vol. 30, no. 8, pp. 1049-1053, https://www.ncbi.nlm.nih.gov/pubmed/17702275

9   James J & Rogers, P 2005, 'Effects of caffeine on performance and mood: withdrawal reversal is the most plausible explanation', *Psychopharmacology*, vol. 182, no. 1, pp. 1-8, https://www.ncbi.nlm.nih.gov/pubmed/16001109

10   Randolph, D & O'Conner P 2017, 'Stair walking is more energizing than lose dose caffeine in sleep deprived young women', *Physiology & Behavior*, vol. 174, pp. 128-135, https://www.ncbi.nlm.nih.gov/pubmed/28302573

11   Yoto, A, Motoki, M, Murao, S & Yokogoshi, H 2012, 'Effects of L-theanine or caffeine intake on changes in blood pressure under physical and psychological stresses', *Journal of Physiological Anthropology*, vol. 31, no.1, pp. 1-9, https://www.ncbi.nlm.nih.gov/pmc/articles/PMC3518171/

12   Sissons, C 2018, 'What are the health benefits of bullet-proof coffee?', *Medical News Today*, https://www.medicalnewstoday.com/articles/323253.php

13   Price, A 2017, 'Is mushroom coffee even better than regular coffee?', *Dr Axe*, https://draxe.com/mushroom-coffee/

14   The World's Healthiest Foods 2017, *Vitamin C*, http://www.whfoods.com/genpage.php?tname=nutrient&dbid=109.

15   Patak, P, Willenberg, H & Bornstein, S 2004, 'Vitamin C is an important cofactor for both adrenal cortex and adrenal medulla', *Endocrine Research*, vol. 30, no. 4, pp. 871-875, https://www.ncbi.nlm.nih.gov/labs/articles/15666839/.

16   Depeint, F, Bruce, W, Shangari, N, Mehta, R & O'Brien, P 2006, 'Mitochondrial function and toxicity: role of the B vitamin family on mitochondrial energy metabolism', *Chemico-Biological Interactions*, vol. 163, no. 1-2, pp. 94-112, https://www.ncbi.nlm.nih.gov/pubmed/16765926

17   Stevenson, S 2016, *Sleep Smarter: 21 essential strategies to sleep your way to a better body, better health and bigger success*, Hay House, New Delhi.

18   Mayo Clinic 2018, *Exercise and stress: Get moving to manage stress*, https://www.mayoclinic.org/healthy-lifestyle/stress-management/in-depth/exercise-and-stress/art-20044469

19   Anderson, E & Shivakumar, G 2013, 'Effects of exercise and physical activity on anxiety', *Frontiers in Psychiatry*, vol. 4, no. 27, https://www.ncbi.nlm.nih.gov/pmc/articles/PMC3632802/

20   Hill, E, Zack, E, Battaglini, C, Viru, M, Viru, A & Hackney A 2008, 'Exercise and circulating Cortisol levels: The intensity threshold effect', *Journal of Endocrinological Investigation*', vol. 31, no. 7, pp. 587-591, https://www.ncbi.nlm.nih.gov/pubmed/18787373

A Depleted and Burnt-Out Immune System

1   Asif, N, Iqbal, R & Nazir, C 2017, 'Human immune system during sleep', *American Journal of Clinical and Experimental Immunology*, vol. 6, no. 6, pp. 92-96, https://www.ncbi.nlm.nih.gov/pubmed/29348984

2   Foster, R 2013, 'Why we sleep', TED Global, https://www.ted.com/talks/russell_foster_why_do_we_sleep?language=en

3   Oliveira de Almeida, C & Malheiro, A, 'Sleep, immunity and shift workers: A review', *Sleep Science*, vol. 9, no. 3, pp. 164-168, https://www.ncbi.nlm.nih.gov/pmc/articles/PMC5241621/

4   Vgontzas, A, Zoumakis, E, Bixler, E, Lin, H, Follett, H, Kales, A and Chrousos G 2004, 'Adverse effects of modest sleep restriction on sleepiness, performance, and inflammatory cytokines', *Journal of Clinical Endocrinology and Metabolism*, vol. 89, no. 5, pp. 2119-2126, https://www.ncbi.nlm.nih.gov/pubmed/15126529

5   Shearer, W, Reuben, J and Reuben J 2001, 'Soluble TNF-a receptor 1 and IL-6 plasma levels in humans subjected to the sleep deprivation model of spaceflight', *Journal of Allergy and Clinical Immunology*, vol. 107, no. 1, pp. 165-170, https://www.ncbi.nlm.nih.gov/pubmed/11150007

6   Meier-Ewert, H, Ridker, P, Rifai, N, Regan, M, Price, N, Dinges, D and Mullington, J 2004, 'Effect of sleep loss on C-reactive protein, an inflammatory marker of cardiovascular risk', *Journal of the American college of Cardiology*, vol. 43, no. 4, pp. 678-683, https://www.ncbi.nlm.nih.gov/pubmed/14975482

7   Duhart, J, Leone, M, Paladino, N, Evans, J, Castanon-Cervantes, O, Davidson, A, Golombek, D 2013, 'Suprachiasmatic astrocytes modulate the circadian clock in response to TNF-a', *Journal of Immunology*, vol. 191, no. 9, pp. 1-9, https://www.ncbi.nlm.nih.gov/pmc/articles/PMC3811024/.

8   Kim, T, Jeong, J & Hong, S 2015, 'The impact of sleep and circadian disturbance on hormones and metabolism', *International Journal of Endocrinology*, vol. 2015, pp. 1-9, https://www.hindawi.com/journals/ije/2015/591729/.

9   Ali, T, Choe, J, Awab, A, Wagener, T & Orr, W 2013, 'Sleep, immunity and inflammation in gastrointestinal disorders, *World Journal of Gastroenterology*, vol. 19., no. 48, pp. 9231-9239, https://www.ncbi.nlm.nih.gov/pubmed/24409051

10 Olson, E 2018, 'Lack of sleep: can it make you sick?', *Mayo Clinic*, https://www.mayoclinic.org/diseases-conditions/insomnia/expert-answers/lack-of-sleep/faq-20057757

11 Nutrition Australia 2018, *Nutrition Australia urges Australians to eat more! Vegetables that is.*, http://www.nutritionaustralia.org/national/news/2018/02/nutrition-australia-urges-australians-eat-more-vegetables

12 Myles, I 2014, 'Fast food fever: Reviewing the impacts of the Western diet on immunity', *Nutrition Journal*, vol. 13 no. 61, pp. 1-17, https://www.ncbi.nlm.nih.gov/pmc/articles/PMC4074336/.

13   Rowland, I, Gibson, G, Heinken, A, Scott, K, Swann, J, Thiele, I & Tuohy, K 2018, 'Gut microbiota functions: metabolism of nutrients and other food components', *European Journal of Nutrition*, vol. 57, no. 1, pp. 1-24, https://www.ncbi.nlm.nih.gov/pubmed/28393285

14   Voigt, R, Forsyth, C, Green, S, Mutlu, E, Engen, P, Vitaterna, M, Turek, F & Keshavarzian, A 2014, 'Circadian disorganization alters intestinal microbiota', *PLoS One*, vol. 9, no. 5, pp. 1-17, https://www.ncbi.nlm.nih.gov/pmc/articles/PMC4029760/.

15   Voigt, R, Summa, K, Forsyth, C, Green, S, Engen, P, Naquib, A, Vitaterna, M, Turek, F & Keshavarzian, A 2016, 'The circadian clock mutation promotes intestinal dysbiosis', *Alcoholism: Clinical and Experimental Research*, vol. 40, no. 2, pp. 1331-1338, https://www.ncbi.nlm.nih.gov/pmc/articles/PMC4977829/

16   Tuohy, K, Fava, F & Viola, R 2014, 'The way to a man's heart is through his gut microbiota – dietary pro and prebiotics for the management of cardiovascular risk, *Proceedings of the Nutrition Society*, vol. 73, no. 2, pp. 172-185, https://www.ncbi.nlm.nih.gov/pubmed/24495527

17   Desai, M, Seekatz, A, Koropatkin, N, Kamada, N, Hickey, C, Wolter, M, Pudlo, N, Kitamoto, S, Terrapon, N, Muller, A, Young, V, Henrissat, B, Wilmes, P, Stappenback, T, Nunez, G & Martens, E 2016, 'A dietary fiber-deprived gut microbiota degrades the colonic mucus barrier and enhances pathogen susceptibility', *Cell*, vol. 167, no. 5, pp. 1339-1353, https://www.ncbi.nlm.nih.gov/pubmed/27863247

18   Koutsos, A, Tuohy, K & Lovegrove, J 2015, 'Apples and cardiovascular health – is the gut microbiota a core consideration?', *Nutrients*, vol. 7, no. 6, pp. 3959-3998, https://www.ncbi.nlm.nih.gov/pmc/articles/PMC4488768/

19   Ahmed, E 2012, 'Exercise and Immunity', *Journal of Novel Physiotherapies*, vol. 2, no. 4, https://www.omicsonline.org/open-access/exercise-and-immunity-2165-7025.1000e115.pdf

20   Nieman, D 2015, 'Moderate exercise improves immunity and decreases illness rates', *American Journal of Lifestyle Medicine*, vol. 5, no. 4, pp. 338-345, https://www.researchgate.net/publication/254075198_Moderate_Exercise_Improves_Immunity_and_Decreases_Illness_Rates

21   Costa, R, Snipe, R, Kitic, C & Gibson, P 2017, 'Systematic review: exercise-induced gastrointestinal syndrome-implications for health and intestinal disease', *Alimentary Pharmacology & Therapeutics*, vol. 46, no. 3, pp. 246-265, https://www.ncbi.nlm.nih.gov/pubmed/28589631

22   Scrivens, D 2008, 'Rebounding: Good for the lymph system', *Well Being Journal*, vol. 17, no. 3, https://www.wellbeingjournal.com/rebounding-good-for-the-lymph-system/

23   Cogoli, A 1991, 'Changes observed in lymphocyte behavior during gravitational unloading', *American Society for Gravitational and Space Biology*, vol. 4, no. 2, pp. 107-115, https://www.ncbi.nlm.nih.gov/pubmed/11537173

24   Cancer Tutor 2017, *Rebounding: Science behind the 7 major health benefits of rebound exercise*, https://www.cancertutor.com/rebounding/

A Disrupted Family and Social Life

1   Guadagni, V, Burles, F, Ferrara, M & Iaria, G 2014, 'The effects of sleep deprivation on emotional empathy', *Journal of Sleep Research*, vol. 23, no. 6, pp. 657-663, https://www.ncbi.nlm.nih.gov/pubmed/25117004

2   Keller, P, Haak, E, DeWall, C & Renzetti, C 2017, 'Poor sleep is associated with greater marital aggression: The role of self-control', *Behavioral Sleep Medicine*, vol. 17, no. 2, pp. 174-180, https://www.tandfonline.com/doi/abs/10.1080/15402002.2017.1312404

3   Krizan, Z & Hisler, G 2018, 'Sleepy anger: Restricted sleep amplifies angry feelings', *Journal of Experimental Psychology: General*, https://www.ncbi.nlm.nih.gov/pubmed/30359072

4   Atkinson, G, Fullick, S, Grindey, C, Maclaren, D & Waterhouse, J 2008, 'Exercise, energy balance and the shift worker', *Sports Medicine*, vol. 38, no. 8, pp. 671-685, https://www.ncbi.nlm.nih.gov/pubmed/18620467

5   Chapman, G 2010, *The 5 Love Languages*, Northfield Publishing, Chicago.

6   White, L & Keith, B 1990, 'The effect of shift work on the quality and stability of marital relations', *Journal of Marriage and the Family*, vol. 52, no. 2, pp. 453-462, http://psycnet.apa.org/record/2001-05384-014

7   Holt-Lunstad, J, Smith, T, Baker, M, Harris, T & Stephenson, D 2015, 'Loneliness and social isolation as risk factors for mortality: a meta-analytic review', *Perspectives of Psychological Science*, vol. 10, no. 2, pp. 227-237, https://journals.sagepub.com/doi/abs/10.1177/1745691614568352?journalCode=ppsa

Healthy Shift Worker Recipes

1   Candice Bauer, registered nurse and co-founder of BAREbyBauer, https://www.barebybauer.com.au/

2   Bailey, C 2016, *The Gut Health Diet Plan*, Watkins Media Limited, London.

3   Mary-Leigh Scheerhorn, clinical nutritionist and founder of Genesis Health and Lifestyle Solutions, https://www.genesishealthandlifestyle.com/

4   Lara Busch, clinical nutritionist and founder of Authentic Nutrition by Lara, https://www.facebook.com/Authentic-Nutrition-BY-LARA-140487806376045/

5   Sara Capacci, degree qualified in complementary medicine and founder of The Connection Project, https://www.theconnectionproject.com.au/

About Audra Starkey

Audra Starkey is a clinically trained nutritionist, accredited trainer, shift work veteran, and founder of *The Healthy Shift Worker* podcast.

After more than twenty years in the aviation industry, Audra decided to switch careers and complete a bachelor of health science degree, majoring in nutritional medicine, to gain a better understanding of the impact circadian rhythm disruption and poor dietary habits have on our health.

With a particular interest in preventative health, she went on to found 'The Healthy Shift Worker', a company that provides shift-work-specific wellness services to individuals, along with corporate wellness programs, via her signature Healthy Shift Worker Workplace Wellness Seminars. She is a huge fan of tennis, or more specifically, Roger Federer, and lives in Brisbane with her husband, Dale.

For more information regarding her training programs, along with speaking enquiries, visit www.healthyshiftworker.com or email audra@healthyshiftworker.com